Urticaria - Diagnosis and Management

Edited by Eleni Papakonstantinou

Published in London, United Kingdom

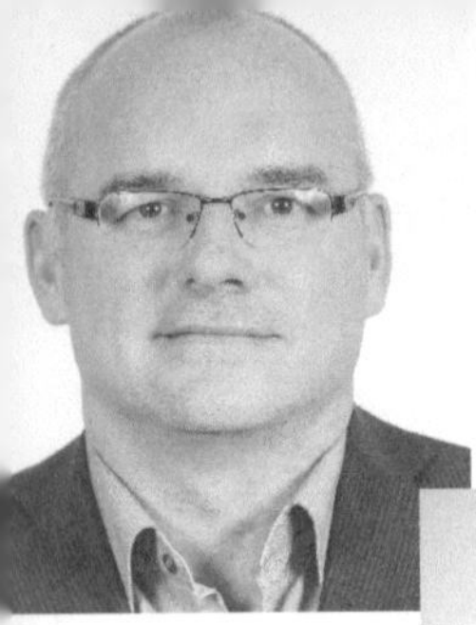
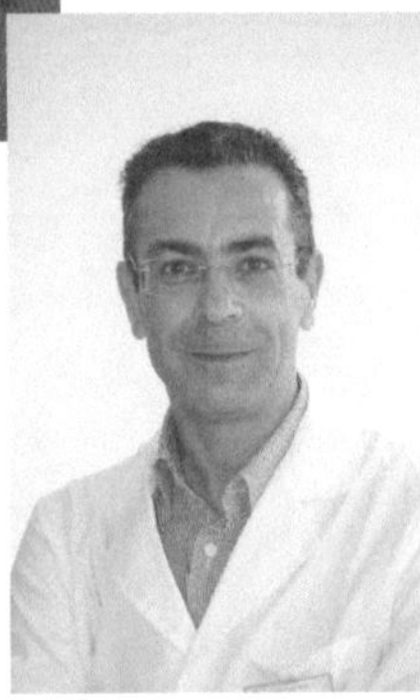
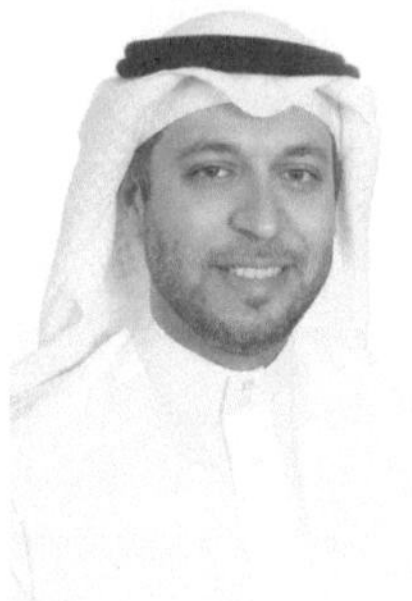
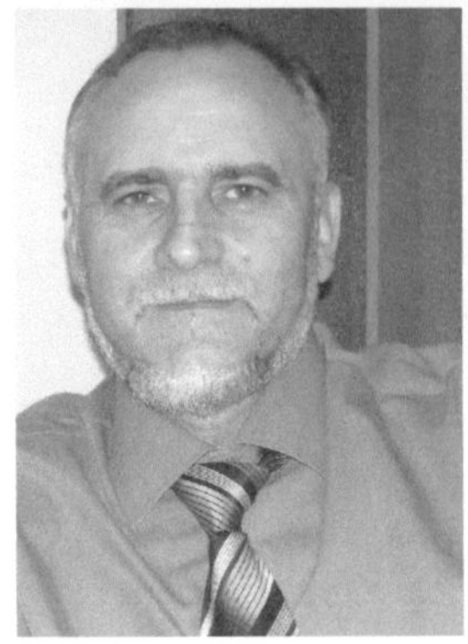
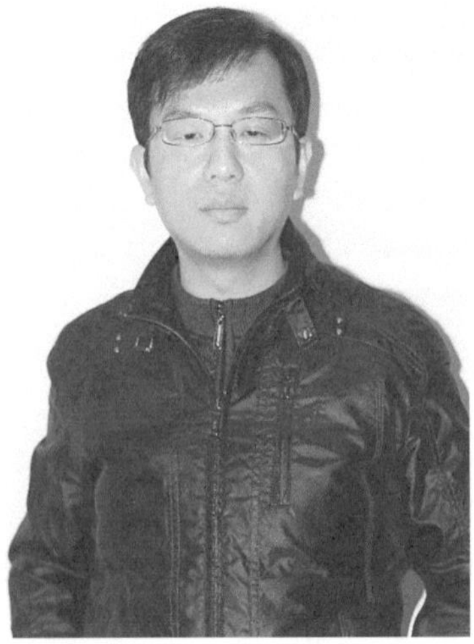
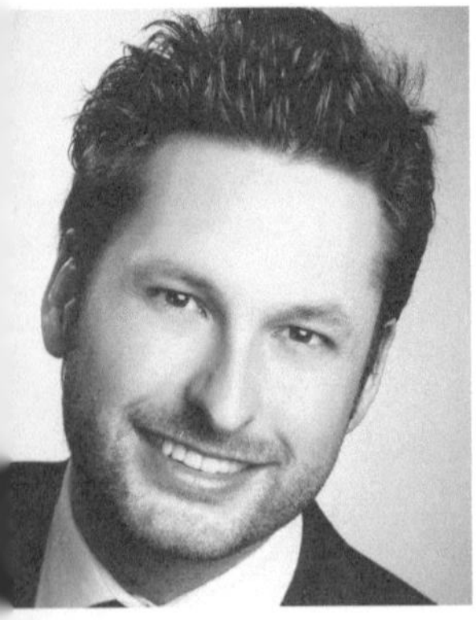
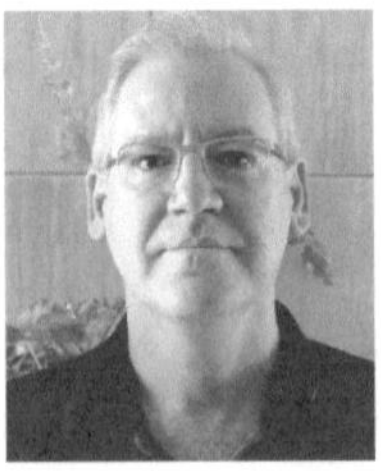

IntechOpen

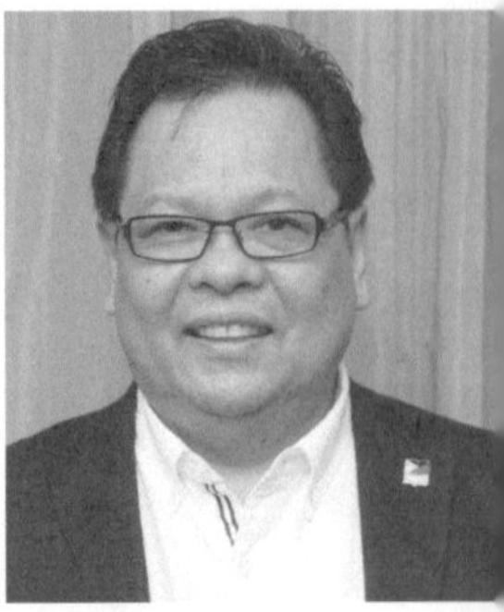
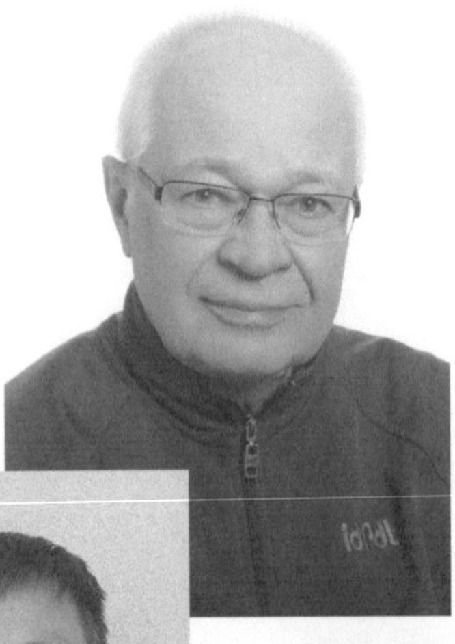
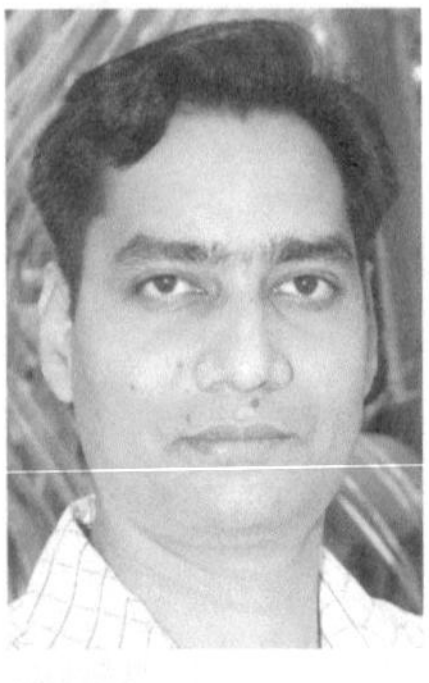
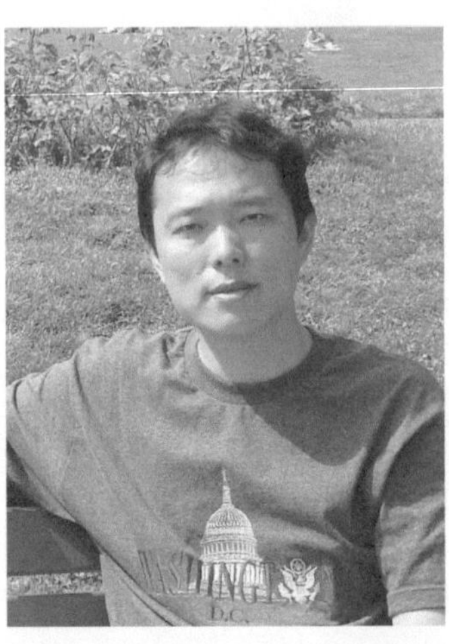
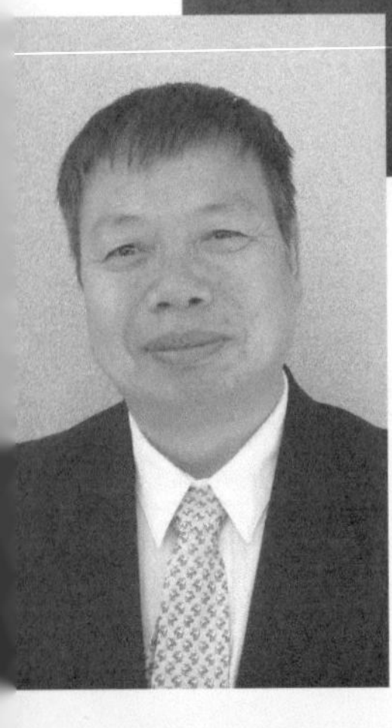
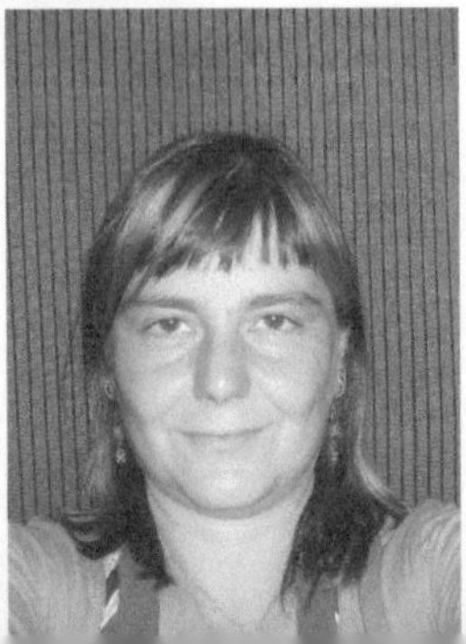

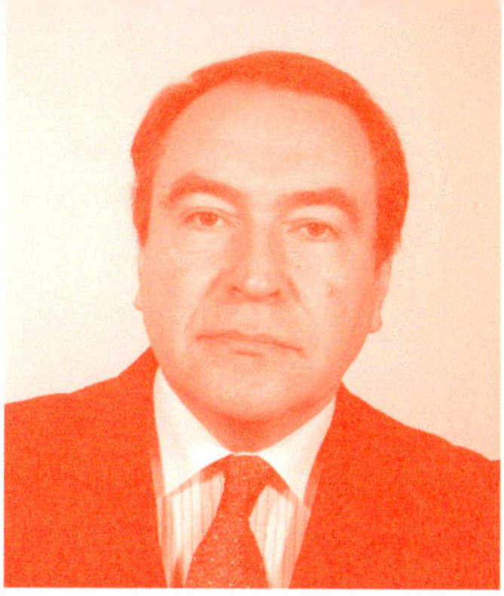
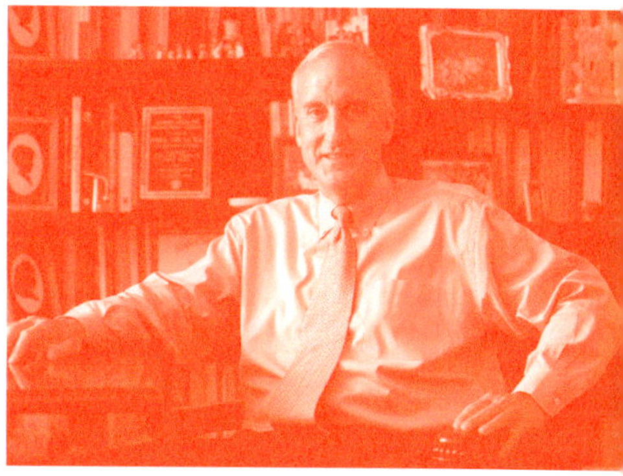
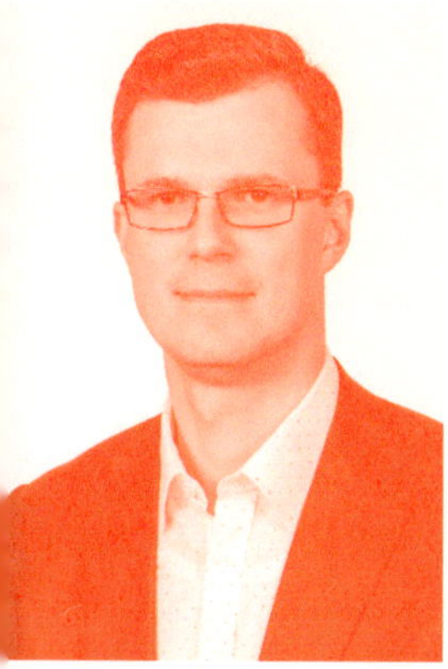
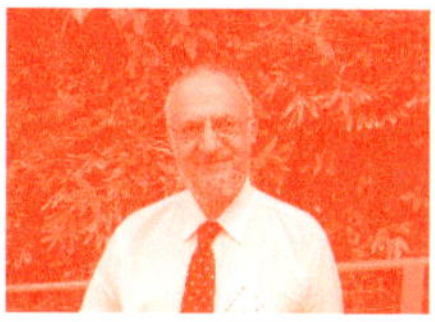
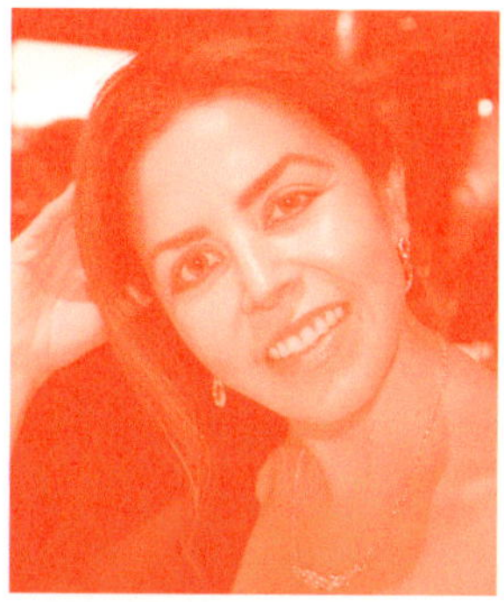

Supporting open minds since 2005

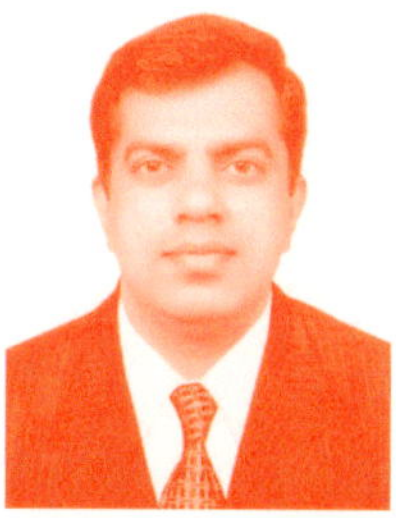
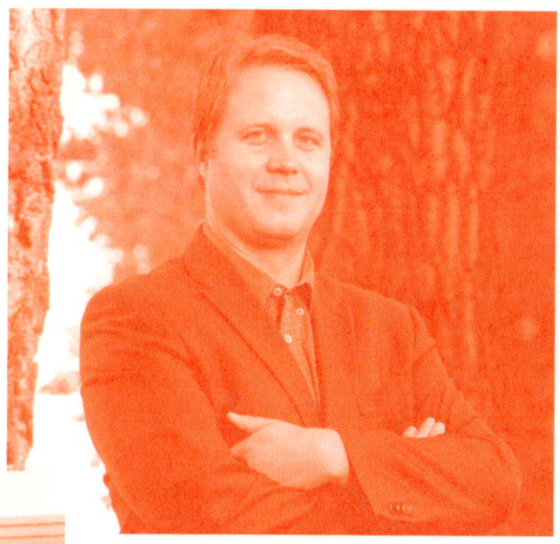
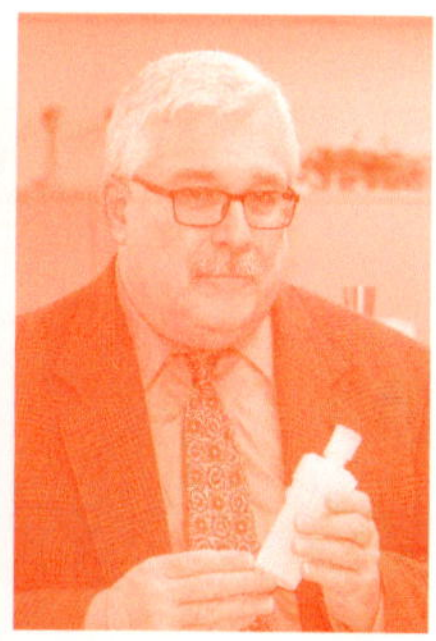
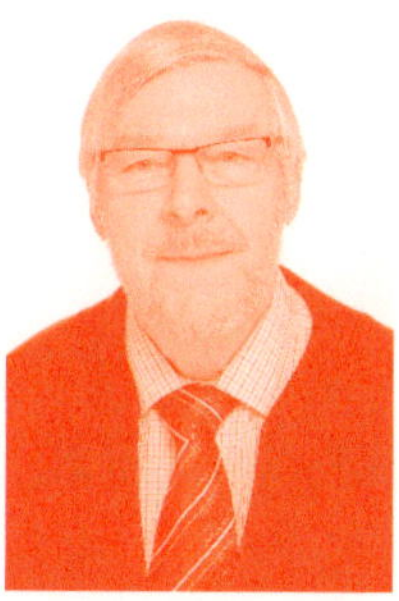
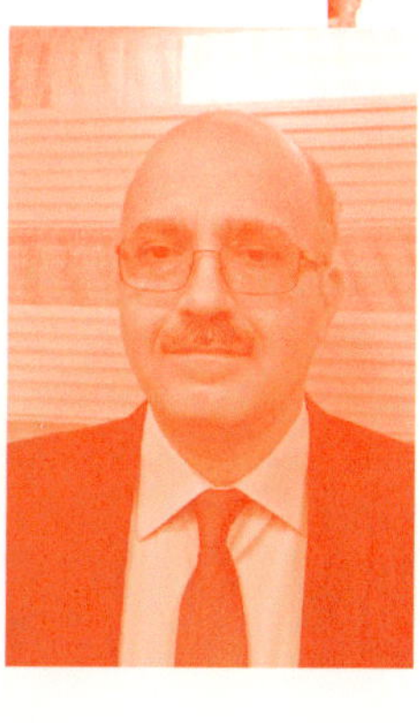
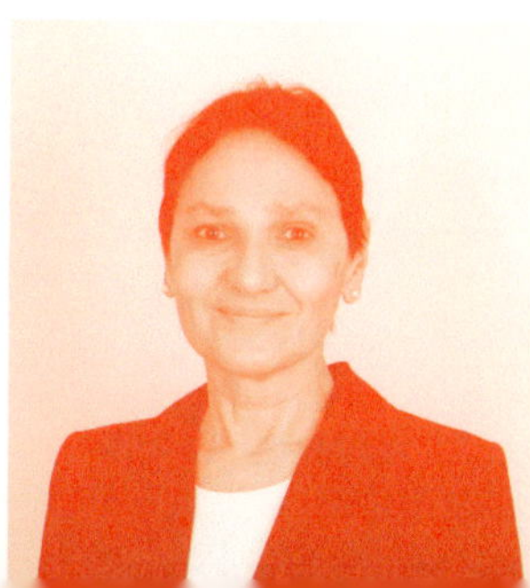
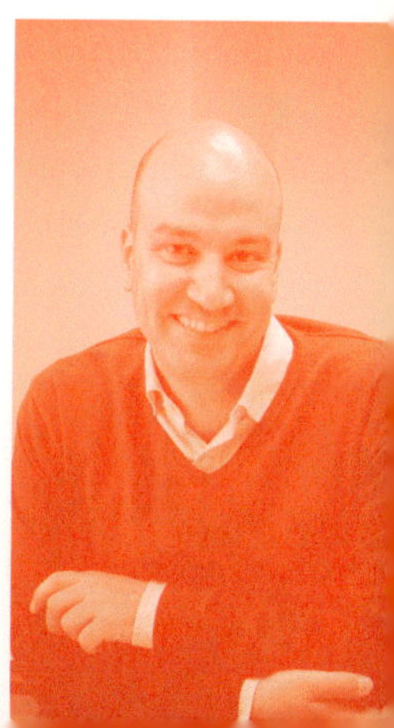

Urticaria - Diagnosis and Management
http://dx.doi.org/10.5772/intechopen.91493
Edited by Eleni Papakonstantinou

Contributors
Evmorfia Ladoyanni, Young-Min Ye, Joaquin Quiralte, María del Robledo Ávila, Stefan Cimbollek, Zahava Vadasz, Elias Toubi, Patrizia Pepe, Victor Desmond Mandel, Eleni Papakonstantinou, Joaquin Quiralte-Castillo

First published in London, United Kingdom, 2021 by IntechOpen
IntechOpen is the global imprint of INTECHOPEN LIMITED, registered in England and Wales, registration number: 11086078, 5 Princes Gate Court, London, SW7 2QJ, United Kingdom
Printed in Croatia

British Library Cataloguing-in-Publication Data
A catalogue record for this book is available from the British Library

Additional hard and PDF copies can be obtained from orders@intechopen.com

Urticaria - Diagnosis and Management
Edited by Eleni Papakonstantinou
p. cm.
Print ISBN 978-1-83969-334-2
Online ISBN 978-1-83969-335-9
eBook (PDF) ISBN 978-1-83969-336-6

Meet the editor

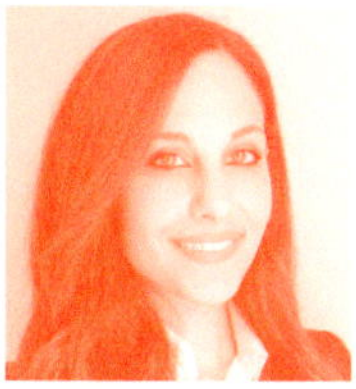

Dr. Eleni Papakonstantinou, MD, is a board-certified dermatologist-venereologist. She studied medicine at the Aristotle University of Thessaloniki, Greece, and continued with her dermatology specialty at the University of Magdeburg and Hannover Medical School, Germany (2012–2017), where she completed her dissertation in 2016 with research work on atopic dermatitis in children. During this time, Dr. Papakonstantinou gained wide experience in the dermatological field with a special focus on the diagnosis and treatment of chronic inflammatory skin diseases and the prevention and treatment of melanocytic and non-melanocytic skin tumors. Her research interests include atopic dermatitis, pruritus, and the pathophysiology of blistering dermatoses. In addition to lectures at national and international congresses, Dr. Papakonstantinou has published more than thirty scientific papers in international medical journals and her work has been recognized with various prizes (poster prize of the German Dermatological Society, Leipzig, 2016), the Michael Hornstein Memorial Scholarship (EADV Athens 2016), and a travel grant (EAACI Vienna, 2016). Since 2017, she has been a specialist dermatologist-venereologist in Germany and a fellow of the European Board of Dermatology-Venereology (FEBDV). She is currently working as a specialist dermatologist in a dermatological practice in Dortmund, Germany, and she co-administrates an international dermatologic network, Wikiderm International, which is an online learning platform presenting news from the world of dermatology.

Contents

Preface XI

Chapter 1 1
Introductory Chapter: Urticaria - Meeting the Diagnostic and Therapeutic Challenge
by Eleni Papakonstantinou

Chapter 2 5
Chronic Spontaneous Urticaria – Diagnosis and Management
by Evmorfia Ladoyanni

Chapter 3 25
Clinical Phenotypes in NSAID-Induced Urticaria/Angioedema
by Joaquin Quiralte, María del Robledo Ávila, Stefan Cimbollek and Joaquin Quiralte-Castillo

Chapter 4 39
The Use of Omalizumab in Chronic Urticaria: Available Data and Future Aspects of Anti-IgE Treatment
by Young-Min Ye

Chapter 5 55
The Role of Anti-IgE Antibodies in Urticaria
by Patrizia Pepe and Victor Desmond Mandel

Chapter 6 95
New Biological Treatment Options in CSU
by Zahava Vadasz and Elias Toubi

Preface

Urticaria is one of the most common dermatological cutaneous reactions. Although it can be easily recognized by patients and physicians, determining its causes, clinical manifestations, and treatment remains challenging.

This book is a practical guide to all types and aspects of urticaria important to physicians. It includes current guidelines and recent literature. Followed by the Introductory chapter, in Chapter 2, Dr. Evmorfia Ladoyanni presents current knowledge about pathophysiology with a focus on the clinically relevant aspects of diagnosis and treatment of the disease. In Chapter 3, Dr. Joaquin Quiralte comprehensively reviews a common type of urticaria caused by nonsteroidal anti-inflammatory drugs, a condition that is challenging to diagnose as well as manage. In Chapters 4 and 5, Prof. Young-Min Ye and Dr. Patrizia Pepe place special emphasis on the management and therapy of urticaria, especially the role of anti-IgE-antibodies. Finally, in Chapter 6, Prof. Zahava Vadasz discusses new biological treatment options for urticaria as well as potential future treatments.

This practical guide is a useful resource for all physicians specializing in dermatology, allergy, internal medicine, pediatrics, and general medicine and offers invaluable assistance in the daily practical management of urticaria patients.

Dr. Eleni Papakonstantinou
Private Dermatological Practice - Hautärzte am Markt,
Dortmund, Germany

Chapter 1

Introductory Chapter: Urticaria - Meeting the Diagnostic and Therapeutic Challenge

Eleni Papakonstantinou

1. Introduction

Urticaria is one of the most common pruritic skin diseases which is characterized by the occurence of recurrent erythematous and edematous wheals with or without angioedema. These wheals appear at different body areas and dissapear within 24 hours while new lesions may occur. The disease may be characterized as idiopathic or inducible depending on the potential trigger factors and acute or chronic depending on the duration of the symptoms for less or more than 6 weeks [1].

The lifetime prevalence of chronic urticaria is about 10–20%. Urticaria can occur at any age but the chronic form is more common in adults, especially during the third and fourth decade of life. The disease can affect both women and men but there is evidence of a female predominance [2].

The pathomechanismus of urticaria is based in the release of various mediators due to degranulation of activated subepidermal mast cells. Released histamine causes local vasodilation and increased capillary permeability, resulting in intracutaneous (wheal) or subcutaneous (angioedema) edema. Furthermore, activation of sensory nerves leads to pruritus and reflex erythema. The mast cell degranulation may be caused by different mechanisms such as direct activation or IgE-mediated allergic activation and results to the release of mediators such as histamin, which is responsible for the pruritus which ist he main symptom in urticaria. Beside pruritus, these vasoactive mediators are responsible for vasodilation and subsequent erythema and edema [3].

Chronic urticaria can be characterized as spontaneous when no trigger factors are known or as inducible when the appearance of wheals is caused by specific trigger factors. There are many triggering factors for chronic urticaria but determining a specific cause is not always possible.

The most common ones include viral, bacterial or parasitic infections, specific drugs (e.g. nonsteroidal anti-inflammatory drugs and antibiotics), foods, physical factors (such as pressure, exposure to light, heat or cold, vibration, exercise and increased body temperature) and emotional stress [4]. Furthermore, autoimmune and systemic diseases and also malignancies can be the underlying factor of urticaria and should be taken into consideration in the diagnosis of the disease. Some of the most common systemic disorders involved in urticaria are lupus erythematosus, cutaneous vasculitis, Sjögren's syndrome, autoimmune thyroid disease, rheumatoid arthritis and diabetes mellitus [5]. All these factors and conditions will be thoroughly disscussed in this book giving the reader a complete guideline to diagnose and define different types of urticaria.

 IntechOpen

Diagnosis of urticaria is mainly based on anamnesis and clinical examination of the patient. However, due to the transient character of the skin manifestations this may be difficult at the time of examination. Sometimes, photos or re-examination of he patient when the lesions are present are necessary and helpful for the clinician in order to make the diagnosis. Thorough clinical history and a potential association with angioedema and/or anaphylaxis should always be asked.

Clinical manifestation of urticaria is characteristic with circumscribed wheals in any region of the body which commonly persist no longer than 24 hours and reappear at different body areas. Pruritus is the major symptom patients claim for which affects their daily activities and quality of life. If the lesions persist longer than 24 hours, appear in combination with skin manifestations such as petechia or hyperpigmentation, or are accombanied by systemic symptoms such as fever and arthralgia, more severe conditions such as urticaria vasculitis have to be excluded with a skin biopsy.

Skin biopsy can be helpful if systemic diseases such are vasculitis or mastocytosis are suspected. Histopathological findings of urticaria include interstitial edema and perivascular mixed cellular infiltrate. T-lymphocytes are predominant in this infiltrate but also eosinophils, neutrophils, and basophils may also be present.

Once the diagnosis is confirmed, it is important to find out potential trigger factors, if possible. Detailed anamnesis is important to determine any triggering infection, drugs or physical factor. Challenge tests may be then individually performed to confirm the different types of inducible urticaria.

Skin tests such as an autologous serum test may be useful in order to exclude the autoimmune type of urticaria. During this test patient's own serum is intradermally injected on the forearm oft he patient and is positiv if an urticarial reaction appears within 30 min.

Laboratory tests are in general not indicated for patients with acute urticaria unless they have signs and symptoms suggesting an underlying systemic disease. In cases of chronic urticaria besides a standard laboratory examination additional tests such as antinuclear antibody, autoantibodies, rheumatoid factor, complement C_3 and C_4 levels, thyroid parameters, Helicobacter pylori antigen, hepatitis and parasite examination are essential in ordert to exclude an infection or an underlying autoimmune disease [1, 6].

The severity of the disease can be individual evaluated using some scoring systems used for this purpose, one of which is the urticaria activity score (UAS). This is a widely used scoring system questioning the intensity of pruritus and the number of wheals in a day and can be further used to also evaluate the effectivity of the therapy in later stages [7].

If an association with trigger factors has been established, the prevention of trigger is the first step of treatment. The next step includes drugs in order to control the symptoms with minimal side effects. Second-generation H_1 antihistamines, such as cetirizine and loratadine, are used as first-line treatment options. These newer, antihistamines ahave a non-sedative character compared to the first-generation ones such as hydroxyzine and diphenhydramine and thus are mopstly preffered. In severe cases, a dose increasement up to fourfold of standard therapeutic doses is recommended by the latest guidelines. In certain cases, H_2 antihistamines may be used in combination with H_1 antihistamines.

Glucocortikosteroids may be used for a short period of time and at the lowest dose in addition to antihistamines for acute urticarial attacks, particularly when accompanied by angioedema. Long-term use of systemic glucocorticoids is not recommended because of potential adverse effects.

In chronic cases where the symptoms persist despite high-dose antihistamines. Antileukotrienes, such as montelukast, zafirlukast as well as the

5-lipoxygenase-inhibitor zileuton are added to antihistamines as second-line treatment options. Furthermore, immunosuppressive agents, such as cyclosporine, are effective in the treatment of chronic urticaria but the clinicians and the patients should be aware of the potential side effects. Other less used drugs such as dapsone, hydroxychloroquine, sulfasalazine, azathioprin and mycophenolate have also been used in the treatment of urticaria [1].

Biologic agents such as omalizumab has recently been added in the treatment of chronic urticaria in adults and adolescents that continue to be symptomatic despite the use H1 antihistamines. It is an anti-IgE monoclonal antibody which has a good efficacy and safety profile in most oft he patients and can be easily applied with monthly subcutaneous injections [8]. Further research is being made and current data indicate ligelizumab, a next-generation anti-IgE antibody as a potential valid alternative for patients with chronic urticaria unresponsive to omalizumab. Other IgE-antibodies and diverse anti-IL factors are also being studied and may show a potential role in the treatment of urticaria [9].

2. Conclusion

In view of the pathomechanism and the different forms of urticaria, the treatment of the disease is a real concern over the opportunities and therapeutic options already available and over all other strategies under development and trials. In this context, it is believed that we will be able personalize the management plan of urticaria in the future and we are close the identification of specific biomarkers for different types of the disease which could also be used as monitoring markers.

This book presents the most current knowledge in the diagnosis and management of urticaria. It also examines the scientific aspect of currently available treatments as well as potential new options for managing severe forms of the disease. The different chapters, written by expert authors all over the world, address some of the most important aspects in the diagnosis and management of urticaria.

Author details

Eleni Papakonstantinou
Private Dermatological Practice, Hautärzte am Markt, Dortmund, Germany

*Address all correspondence to: elenipap2000@hotmail.com

References

[1] Zuberbier T, Aberer W, Asero R, et al. The EAACI/GA2LEN/EDF/WAO guideline for the definition, classification, diagnosis, and management of urticaria. Allergy. 2018;73:1393-1414.

[2] Zuberbier T, Balke M, Worm M, Edenharter G, Maurer M. Epidemiology of urticaria: A representative cross-sectional population survey. Clinical and Experimental Dermatology. 2010;35:869-873.

[3] Jain S. Pathogenesis of chronic urticaria: An overview. Dermatology Research and Practice. 2014;2014: 674709.

[4] Abajian M, Schoepke N, Altrichter S, Zuberbier T, Maurer M. Physical urticarias and cholinergic urticaria. Immunol Allergy Clin North Am. 2014;34:73-88.

[5] Davis M, van der Hilst J. Mimickers of urticaria: Urticarial vasculitis and autoinflammatory diseases. J Allergy Clin Immunol Pract. 2018;6:1162-1170.

[6] Maurer M, Fluhr J, Khan D. How to approach chronic inducible urticaria. J Allergy Clin Immunol Pract. 2018;6: 1119-1130.

[7] Hawro T, Ohanyan T, Schoepke N, et al. The urticaria activity score-validity, reliability, and responsiveness. J Allergy Clin Immunol Pract. 2018;6:1185-1190.

[8] Maurer M, Rosén K, Hsieh H, et al. Omalizumab for the treatment of chronic idiopathic or spontaneous urticaria. N Engl J Med. 2013;368: 924-935.

[9] Kocatürk E, Zuberbier T. New biologics in the treatment of urticaria. Curr Opin Allergy Clin Immunol. 2018;18:425-431.

Chapter 2

Chronic Spontaneous Urticaria – Diagnosis and Management

Evmorfia Ladoyanni

Abstract

Chronic urticaria can be subclassified into chronic spontaneous urticaria and chronic inducible urticaria. Up to 30% of cases are associated with functional immunoglobulin G antibodies to the high affinity immunoglobulin E receptor FcεRIα or to immunoglobulin A. Pathogenic activation of mast cells and basophils gives rise to release of pro-inflammatory mediators that lead to development of hives. CSU is a debilitating disease with a relapsing course. It affects 0.5–1% of the population at any given time. The duration of CSU is generally 1–5 years but can be longer in cases associated with angioedema and autoreactivity. CSU has detrimental effects on life quality with sleep-deprivation and psychiatric disorders being the most frequent. In a great number of patients an underlying cause or eliciting factor cannot be identified. Among the patients in which an aetiology is suspected, infections, medication, food and psychological factors are most commonly associated. A potential autoimmune cause has been reported in up to 50% of patients. Chronic inducible urticaria is characterised by its ability to be triggered consistently and reproducibly in response to a specific stimulus (pressure, temperature, vibration, water, heat, light). Antihistamines form the mainstay of therapy. In recalcitrant chronic urticaria, a variety of other drugs have been tried.

Keywords: Wheals, Angioedema, Chronic Spontaneous Urticaria, Chronic Inducible Urticaria, Classification, Prevalence, Histamine-mediated, Pathophysiology, anti-IgE, anti-FcεRI, Autoallergy, anti-TPO, Autoimmune urticaria, Vitamin D, Pseudoallergens, Stress, associated conditions, Predictors of severity, Diagnosis, Medical History, Histopathology, Check List, Clinical signs, Differential Diagnosis, Guidelines, Patient reported outcomes, UAS7, DLQI, Socio-economic burden, Patient characteristics, real-world study, Refractory chronic urticaria, Treatment, Antihistamines, Omalizumab, Leukotriene receptor antagonist, oral corticosteroids

1. Introduction

Chronic urticaria can be subclassified into chronic spontaneous urticaria and chronic inducible urticaria. Up to 30% of cases are associated with functional immunoglobulin G antibodies to the high affinity immunoglobulin E receptor FcεRIα or to immunoglobulin A. Pathogenic activation of mast cells and basophils gives rise to release of pro-inflammatory mediators that lead to development of hives. CSU is a debilitating disease with a relapsing course. It affects 0.5–1% of the population at any given time. The duration of CSU is generally 1–5 years but can be longer in cases associated with angioedema and autoreactivity. CSU has detrimental effects on life quality with sleep-deprivation and psychiatric disorders being the most frequent. In a great number of patients an underlying cause or eliciting factor cannot be identified. Among the patients in which an aetiology is suspected, infections, medication, food and psychological factors are most commonly associated. A potential autoimmune cause has been reported in up to 50% of patients. Chronic inducible urticaria is characterised by its ability to be triggered consistently and reproducibly in response to a specific stimulus (pressure, temperature, vibration, water, heat, light). Antihistamines form the mainstay of therapy. In recalcitrant chronic urticaria a variety of other drugs have been tried that include leukotriene receptor inhibitors, conventional immunosuppressive systemic therapy, anti-inflammatory and biologic therapy. In this chapter we give an overview of CU and CSU in particular and discuss its diagnosis and management.

2. Definition

Urticaria is a relatively common condition that can persist for weeks, months or years and can affect significantly quality of life [1]. It is a heterogenous skin disorder that can be acute or chronic, intermittent or persistent and can occur alone or in association with other related conditions. The aetiology is often difficult to determine particularly in chronic urticaria[1].

Urticaria is characterised by the development of wheals, angioedema or both on the skin [2]. It is characterised by 3 features [3]:

1. Localised erythema and swelling of upper dermal layers

2. Itching and burning sensation of the skin

3. Transient nature – wheal resolves without scarring and skin returns to normal within 1–24 hours

Angioedema [3] is characterised by sudden onset localised swelling of submucosal surfaces of the upper respiratory and gastrointestinal tract, deeper dermal layers of skin including subcutaneous tissue [4]. It is associated more with pain and burning rather than itching and generally takes longer – up to 72 hours - to resolve [3].

Wheals can occur in combination with angioedema in 40% and angioedema can be the only manifestation of urticaria in 20% of patients [1, 5].

Urticaria are classified into 2 major categories [2, 3, 5] – acute vs. chronic – according to duration, and - spontaneous vs. inducible - according to aetiology [5]. Acute urticaria resolves in less than 6 weeks. Chronic urticaria lasts for longer than 6 weeks (**Table 1**).

Many cases of acute urticaria (AU) resolve but 20–45% continue and become chronic [5]. The most common causes for acute urticaria include acute viral infections and allergic reactions to food, medication, latex and insect bites [5, 6].

Chronic urticaria (CU) are clinically subdivided into spontaneous (CSU) - no specific eliciting factor(s) can be identified [7] - and inducible (CINDU) when specific identifiable stimuli trigger urticaria [7].

In summary CSU is characterised by spontaneous occurrence of wheals and or angioedema for 6 or more weeks, resulting from unidentified causes and pathophysiology that is not completely understood [3]. While autoimmune disease (21%), chronic infection (29%), and immune dysfunction (4%) may become evident over

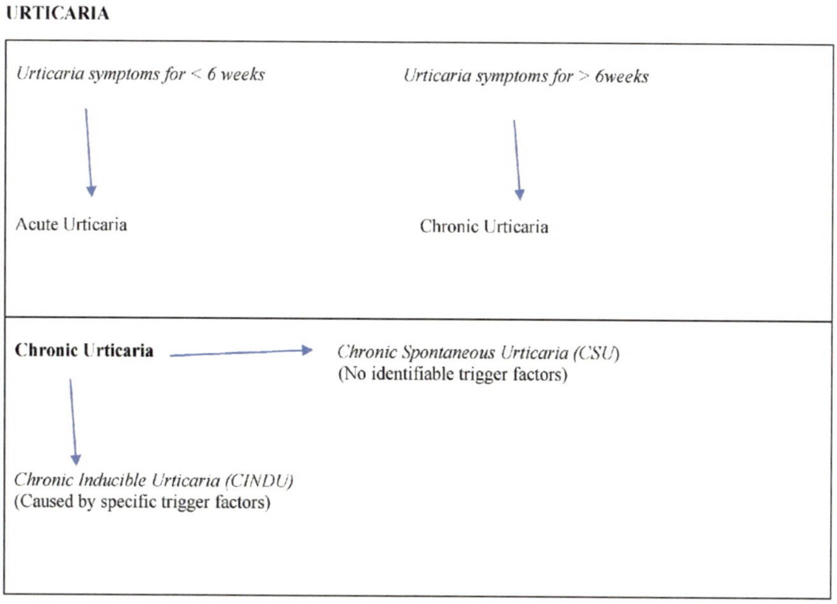

Table 1.
Classification of urticaria [2].

time, in 45% of CSU cases no underlying cause can be found even after 10-year follow-up [4, 5, 8]. In these cases, anaphylaxis does not occur even if angioedema may be present [1, 4].

It is worth mentioning that the term CSU replaced the terms chronic idiopathic urticaria and chronic autoimmune urticaria, whereas the term CINDU replaced the terms physical urticaria and other forms of inducible urticaria, such as cholinergic and aquagenic urticaria [6].

Two or more different subtypes of urticaria may coexist in any given patient. There is often overlap between CSU and CINDU [3, 5].

3. Epidemiology, underlying pathogenesis and trigger factors

3.1 Epidemiology

Evidence suggests [9] that the prevalence of CSU is geographically heterogenous, high in all groups and increasing. It is just as common in children as it is in adults [9]. Lifetime prevalence is 9% [5] with an overall point prevalence in all age groups estimated at 0.7% [4, 9]. The point prevalence is higher in women than in men (1.3% vs. 0.8%) [4, 9] but same in children (1.1% boys vs. 1% girls) [9]. CSU is more common in adolescents and the commonest subgroup of CU [2]. It has a lifetime risk of 20% [7] and is self-limiting with an average duration of 2–5 years, although in up to 30% of patients the symptoms may persist for >5 years [10].

3.2 Underlying pathogenesis

There is little doubt that the release of histamine by mast cells (MC) and basophils represent the final stage in the pathogenesis of CU cases [4]. There is however still uncertainty about the factors that activate these cells and lead to cell degranulation

[11]. Several lines of evidence suggest that different biologic systems like immunity, inflammation and coagulation may contribute to wheal development [4, 11].

There are immunologic and non-immunologic mechanisms that lead to MC degranulation and release of mediators including histamine, leukotrienes and prostaglandins [4, 6]. These mediators recruit basophils, eosinophils, polymononuclear cells and lymphocytes [4, 6] and cause the typical skin manifestations of (a) pruritus via sensory nerve stimulation, (b) vascular dilatation and permeability that leads to extravasation and (c) oedema in upper dermis (wheals) and lower dermis/subcutaneous tissue (angioedema) [6].

The **non-immunologic** pathogenesis involves dysregulation of intracellular signalling pathways within MCs and basophils that lead to defects in trafficking and function of these cells [4]. The immunologic pathway involves the development of autoantibodies to IgE or the high affinity IgE receptor FcεRIα on MCs and basophils [4, 9].

Two types of **immunological CSU** have been identified namely Type I and Type IIb [9]:

- Type I autoimmune CSU is driven by anti-IgE antibodies to autoallergens while

- Type IIb autoimmune CSU is due to autoantibodies that target directly and activate MC degranulation

In type I autoimmune CSU, autoantigens crosslink IgE autoantibodies and bind on MCs and basophils to cause release of vasoactive mediators. Thyroperoxidase (TPO) is the commonest autoallergen binding to IgE (IgE-anti-TPO), other autoantigens include thyroglobulin, tissue factor and IL-24 [4, 9]. Furthermore, some studies have demonstrated that the raised IgE autoantibodies contribute to the increased total serum IgE level found in CSU patients [4, 9].

In type IIb autoimmune CSU, autoantibodies of IgG or IgM type bind to antigen on the target cell (MC) and cause release of mediators. Furthermore, IgG and to a lesser degree IgM and IgA autoantibodies to IgE high affinity receptor FcεRI on MCs and basophils have been identified in roughly 50% of CSU [5, 9]. CSU patients show positive reaction to autologous serum skin test (ASST), that is flare and wheal development to intradermal injection of patient's own serum [4, 9, 12].

Some evidence suggests that type I and IIb autoimmune CSU differ in their clinical features, laboratory markers and response to therapy [9, 13]. Type IIb autoimmune CSU is thought to exhibit higher disease activity, longer duration, higher rates of associated autoimmunity and eosinopenia and basopenia, both markers of recalcitrant disease [9, 13].

CSU is characterised by a **systemic pro-inflammatory state** [11]. Many patients have slightly raised levels of C-reactive protein [8, 13]. Studies [4, 11] also suggest higher association with metabolic syndrome, hyperlipidemia, Multiple sclerosis and other autoimmune conditions (Rheumatoid arthritis, Systemic Lupus Erythematosus) [4, 9].

3.3 Trigger factors

Higher emotional stress is known to contribute to low grade inflammation [8]. Patients with CSU are reported to experience higher rates of anxiety, depression and somatiform disorders [5], although it is unclear if they are cause or effect of CSU [8]. Psychiatric comorbidity has been linked as an additional factor that affects quality of life in CSU patients [5, 12].

Coagulation pathway: Specific studies have demonstrated that the coagulation pathway is activated in CU and involves first the extrinsic pathway followed by the intrinsic pathway. This activation of coagulation pathway is thought to be an intermediate step in CSU pathophysiology [4, 11].

Drugs have been implicated in CU development. The commonest include angiotensin- converting enzyme (ACE) inhibitors and nonsteroidal anti-inflammatory drugs (NSAIDs) [3, 5]. NSAIDs are an aggravating factor in 12–30% of CSU patients [3, 5]. They can also induce urticaria/angioedema in the absence of urticaria history [5]. ACE inhibitor – induced urticaria/angioedema is caused by non-immunologic accumulation of bradykinin and other neurokinins [5] and can occur from weeks to years after ACE inhibitor therapy is commenced.

Food: Type I food allergy is a rare cause of CSU. It should be considered in patients with intermittent symptoms and within 1 hour of exposure to food [5]. The role of food additives as a cause of CSU is unclear. Some studies demonstrated resolution of CSU symptoms after 14 days of pseudoallergen avoidance in up to 30% of patients [5, 8, 14]. Low serum Vitamin D levels and vitamin D supplementation has been reported to improve small numbers of recalcitrant CSU [8, 15].

Infections have been implicated as cause of CSU and include bacterial, viral, parasitic and fungal organisms. Frequency and relevance depend on local population and geographic location [5]. *Anisakis simplex*, a sea fish nematode is relevant in the Mediterranean in the context of CSU [5, 16]. *Helicobacter Pylori* (HP) gastritis has been reported in association with CSU and some studies have reported CSU improvement with HP eradication [3, 5, 8, 17] (**Table 2**).

3.3.1 Contact urticaria

Not all urticaria are mast cell or histamine dependent. Contact urticaria to sorbic acid, methyl nicotinate, cinnamic acid, cinnamic aldehyde and dimethyl sulfoxide are thought to be due to prostaglandins released directly from the epidermis. They do not respond to treatment with antihistamines but improve with salicylic acid and NSAIDs [5].

3.3.2 CINDU

In *CINDU* signs and symptoms usually are elicited by a specific factor and occur in exposed areas that are reproducible by provocation tests [5, 9]. Diagnosis is based on patient history and provocation tests [5] where possible.

Associated Factors that affect prevalence and severity of CSU	
Factor (s)	*Effect (s)*
Autoimmunity	Predisposes to CSU
Food additives/pseudoallergens	Facilitates CSU
Increased stress	Predisposes & Facilitates CSU
Parasitic infection	Predisposes to CSU
Helicobacter Pylori gastritis	Predisposes to CSU
Metabolic Syndrome	Pro-inflammatory state
Low Vitamin D3	Facilitates CSU
Dysbiosis of GI-Tract	Predisposes to CSU

Table 2.
CSU associated factors [8].

Chronic INDuced Urticaria (CINDU) occur when identifiable stimuli trigger urticaria
• Symptomatic Dermographism (mechanical shearing forces, hives arise after 1-5 min) • Cold Urticaria (cold air, cold water, cold wind) • Delayed Pressure Urticaria (vertical pressure, hives arise within 3–8 hours) • Contact Urticaria (urticariogenic substances) • Aquagenic Urticaria (water) • Solar Urticaria (UV and/or visible light) • Heat Urticaria (localised heat) • Vibratory Urticaria/Angioedema (vibratory forces e.g. pneumatic hammer) • Cholinergic Urticaria (by increase of body temperature)
Diagnosis of CINDU is based on clinical history and where possible as result of provocation tests. It is paramount to identify accurately the specific trigger factor, confirm the diagnosis and assess the disease activity.
• Two or more different subtypes of urticaria can coexist in any given patient. • Often there is overlap between CINDU and CSU.

Table 3.
List of different types of CINDU and their associated eliciting factors [5, 7, 10].

Patients can develop systemic signs during provocation testing including nausea, vomiting, diarrhoea, vertigo, wheezing and even anaphylactic shock [5]. CINDU is responsible for 20–30% of all CU and can be associated with CSU in 14–36% (**Table 3**) [2, 4, 5, 9].

4. Diagnosis of urticaria - medical history, clinical signs and symptoms, histopathology, laboratory testing and associated conditions

4.1 Medical history

Urticaria is characterised by the presence of wheals or angioedema. A detailed history and physical examination are essential for correct urticaria diagnosis and appropriate therapy. They help to exclude alternative diagnoses and are guide to what additional investigations are required.

An easy tool checklist for establishing a complete medical history for CU can be seen in **Table 4**.

4.2 Clinical signs and symptoms

CSU is characterised by the onset of pruritic hives and/or angioedema. Hives are well circumscribed areas of non-pitting oedema with blanched centres and raised borders that involve only superficial portion of the dermis and occur with surrounding skin erythema [4]. Wheals can be anywhere on the body and can be distributed widely [2, 5] (**Figure 1**). They can be a few millimetres to several centimetres in diameter, red or white in colour although they are bright red when they flare [4] (**Figures 2** and **3**). They can last from few minutes to several hours, can take any shape or form and can change shape before they resolve. They can be round and form rings or giant patches. They can have a map-like pattern [2]. The wheals tend to resolve in less than 24 hours and can occur at certain times during the day [2]. Hives are more persistent in CSU than CINDU.

Checklist for complete CU Medical History
1. *Time of disease onset: > < 2 hours*
2. *Duration of wheals: > < 24 hours*
3. *Shape, size, colour and distribution of wheals*
4. *Associated Angioedema*
5. *Associated subjective symptoms (itching, pain, burning)*
6. *Diurnal and nocturnal variation*
7. *Occurrence during weekends, holidays or foreign travel*
8. *Family and past medical history of urticaria or atopy*
9. *Past medical history of internal diseases, infections, known allergies*
10. *Psychosomatic and psychiatric disorders*
11. *Gastric or intestinal problems*
12. *Surgical implantation or events during surgery or after local anaesthesia*
13. *Induction by physical stimuli or exercise*
14. *Use of medication (NSAIDs, ACE-inhibitors, immunisations, hormones, laxatives, eye and ear drops, alternative remedies)*
15. *Observed correlation with food intake*
16. *Relationship to menstrual cycle*
17. *Smoking habits (perfumed tobacco products or cannabis)*
18. *Type of work (health care, agriculture, dairy and veterinary work, hairdressers, food handlers, plumbers, packers, painters through exposure to cyclic anhydrites)*
19. *Hobbies*
20. *Stress*
21. *Impact on quality of life by urticaria/angioedema (UAS7, AAS)*
22. *Prior treatment and response to treatment*

Table 4.
Checklist for establishing a complete medical history for CU [2, 3, 5].

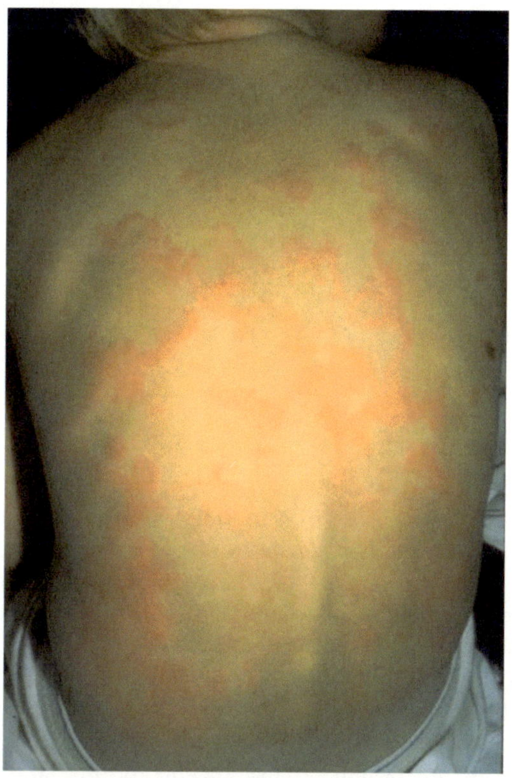

Figure 1.
Widely distributed wheals (courtesy of Dr. Stephen Orpin, Solihull hospital, Birmingham).

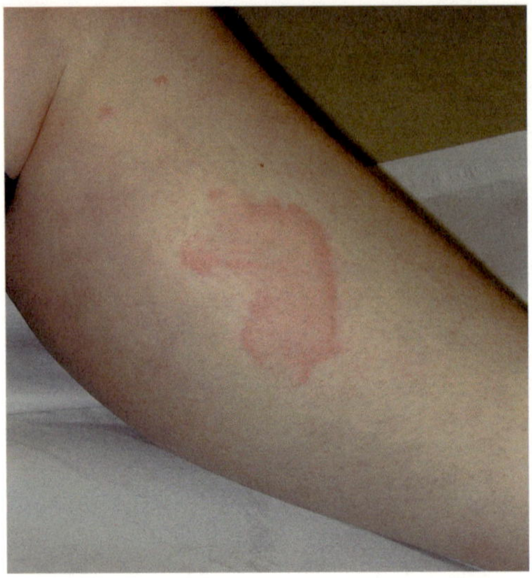

Figure 2.
Solitary wheal (courtesy of Dr. Stephen Orpin, Solihull hospital, Birmingham).

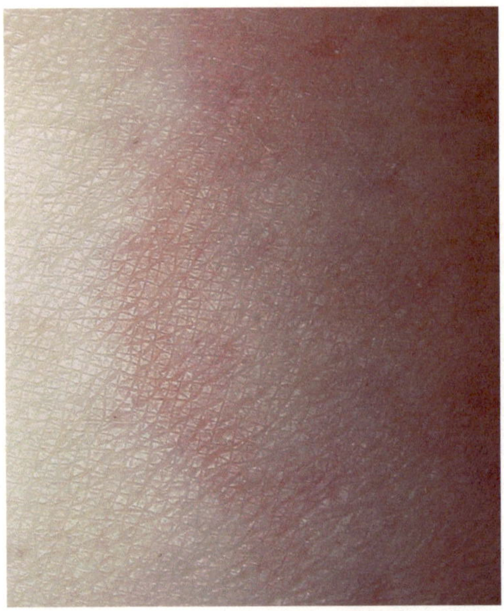

Figure 3.
Solitary wheal in higher power (courtesy of Dr. Stephen Orpin, Solihull hospital, Birmingham).

Dermographism (**Figures 4** and **5**) is inducible and comprises of wheal development when the skin is stroked. It can occur on its own but also in the context of CSU and CINDU. When elicited it can support the diagnosis of urticaria.

Angioedema is more often localised and commonly affects the face in perioral and periorbital distribution, the lips, tongue, eyelids, hands, feet, genitalia and rarely bowel [2, 5]. Lesions tend to be fainter in colour and often painful (**Figure 6**). It can occur in combination with wheals.

Up to 16% of CU patients can experience systemic symptoms during a flare [5]. Systemic symptoms include fatigue, arthralgia and abdominal pain (30%), but also headache, myalgia, retrosternal oppression, wheezing, dyspnoea, rhinorrhoea, flushing, palpitations, and ocular irritation [2, 5, 16].

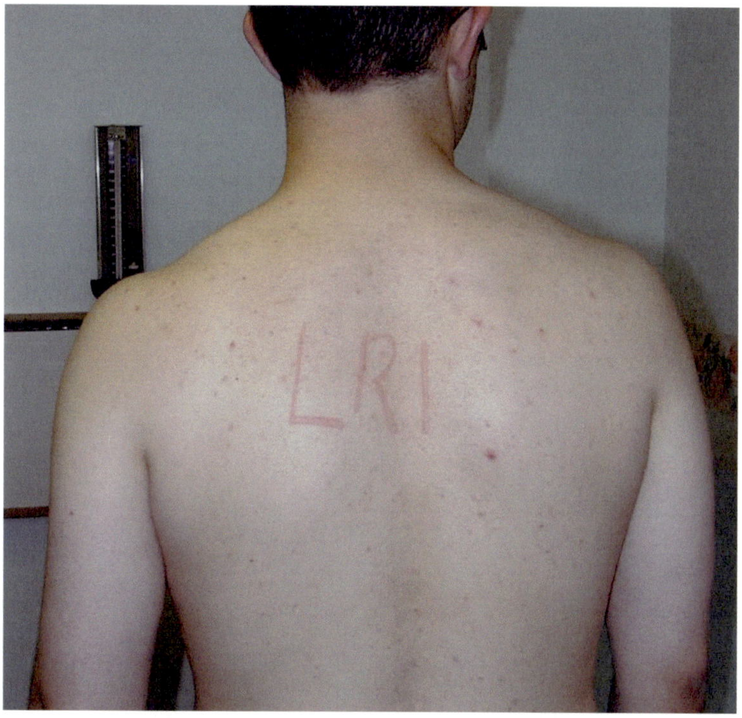

Figure 4.
Dermographism (courtesy of Dr. Stephen Orpin, Solihull hospital, Birmingham).

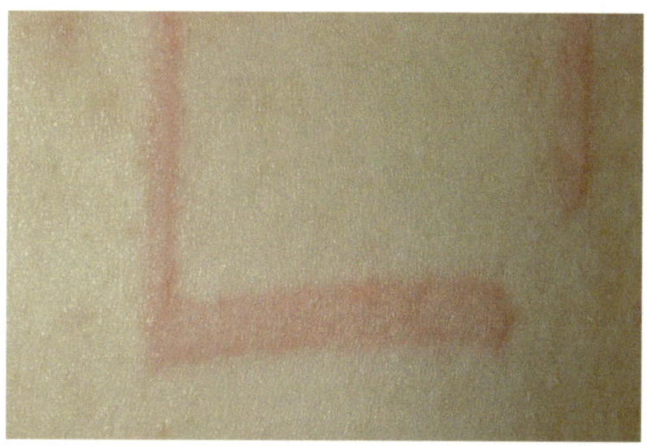

Figure 5.
Dermographism - higher power (courtesy of Dr. Stephen Orpin, Solihull hospital, Birmingham).

Physical examination should include assessment of skin [2, 5, 8, 9] for:

- the presence of wheals and angioedema
- provocation of dermographism
- any signs of purpura
- evaluation of residual lesions in areas hard to reach for patient (urticarial vasculitis)
- any signs of any underlying and/or associated conditions.

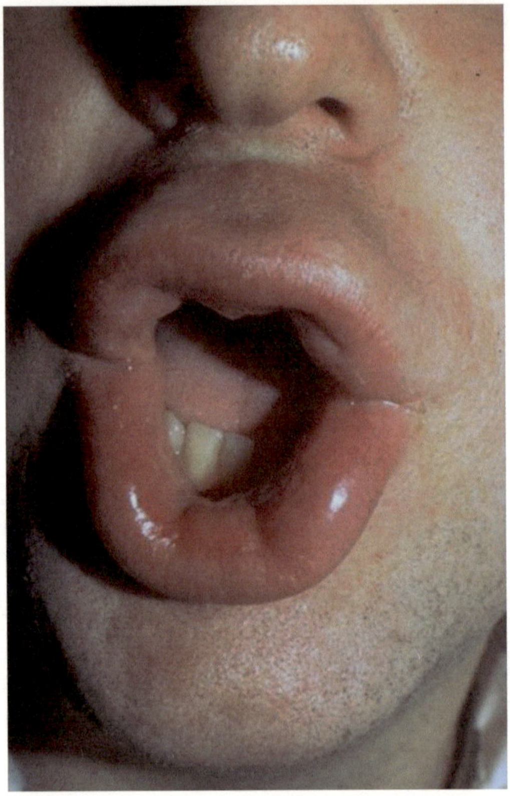

Figure 6.
Angioedema of lips (courtesy of Dr. Stephen Orpin, Solihull hospital, Birmingham).

Conditions that are associated with urticaria +/– angioedema
Syndromes presenting with urticaria +/– angioedema: • Cryopyrin – associated periodic syndromes including familial autoinflammatory syndrome • Muckle - Wells syndrome • Neonatal – onset multisystem inflammatory disease • Chronic infantile neurologic, cutaneous and articular syndrome • Schnitzler syndrome • Gleich syndrome • Phospholipase Cg2 – associated antibody deficiency
Diseases related to urticaria: • Urticarial Vasculitis • Serum-sickness like reaction • Bradykinin-mediated angioedema including hereditary angioedema and ACE-inhibitor induced angioedema • Urticaria Pigmentosa (Maculopapular Cutaneous Mastocytosis) • Bullous Pemphigoid (during pre-bullous stage) • Exercise induced anaphylaxis • Antropod bites
Hives are not always itchy and are often flatter in appearance

Table 5.
Diseases that can present with urticarial lesions [2, 5].

4.3 Histopathology

Histopathologic findings are usually mild and include sparse perivascular and interstitial mixed inflammatory infiltrate and upper dermal oedema [5]. If vascular damage is present urticarial vasculitis (UV) needs to be excluded. UV affects the superficial vascular dermal plexus and shows subtle features of leucocytoclastic vasculitis [5].

4.4 Laboratory testing and associated conditions

The diagnosis of CU is often made on clinical grounds, a limited routine diagnostic work-up is recommended in a case-by-case basis [5, 8]. A skin biopsy should be considered in patients that do not respond to H1 antihistamines, and when an alternative diagnosis is considered (**Table 5**) [5].

5. Disease activity scores used in chronic urticaria and burden of disease

5.1 Disease activity scores used in chronic urticaria

CSU affects several domains of health-related quality of life, such as daily living, sleep, emotional and psychological well-being as well as work productivity [9, 18]. Several types of patient-reported-outcome (PRO) instruments have been used to assess quality of life and disease burden in CSU. They include:

- ED-5D (generic)
- Dermatology Life Quality Index (DLQI) (generic dermatological)
- Disease-specific Chronic Urticaria Quality of Life Questionnaire (CU-Q2oL)
- Angioedema Quality of Life Questionnaire (AE-QoL)
- Urticaria Activity Score (UAS) (**Table 6**)
- Angioedema Activity Score (AAS)
- Urticaria Control Test (UCT)

The inclusion of PRO instruments in clinical practice is increasingly recommended by clinicians and commissioners as it allows patient input and view of their disease

The Weekly Urticaria Activity Score (UAS7)	
Wheals Score	*Pruritus Score*
0 = No wheals	0 = None
1 = Mild (< 20 wheals)	1 = Mild (present but not annoying or troublesome)
2 = Moderate (20–50 wheals)	2 = Moderate (troublesome but does not interfere with normal daily activity or sleep)
3 = Intense (>50 wheals)	3 = Intense (severe itch, which is sufficiently troublesome to interfere with normal daily activity or sleep)

Table 6.
UAS7 = score for hives + score for itch = daily score; repeat daily assessments for 7 days and add up daily scores for UAS7 [2, 18].

and response to therapy and can contribute to better informed treatment decisions and improve physician-patient communication.

The UAS (**Table 6**) is a diary-based PRO measure that assesses the key sign hives and the key symptom itch of CU. The international EAACI/GA^{2}LEN/EDF/WAO guidelines for urticaria recommend the use of UAS in clinical practice to determine disease activity and response to treatment [9, 13, 18]. The UAS is calculated as the sum of the daily number of wheals and the pruritus severity score over a period of 7 days (UAS7). Currently two versions exist of the daily UAS7 – in the first version patients score themselves once per day (every 24 hours), in the second version the scoring happens twice daily (every 12 hours). No significant difference [18] has been identified between the two versions. It is recommended that the same version be used consistently in the same patient in order to be able to evaluate the results [16]. In current clinical practice most use the once daily scoring version, as it is less burdensome for patients. The Urticaria Control Test (UCT) is a retrospective tool consisting of four questions with a clear cut-off scoring for "well-controlled" vs. "poorly controlled" [6].

In regular clinical practice the PRO instruments commonly used to assess CU disease activity, disease control and effects on quality of life include the UAS7 and the DLQI [2].

5.2 Burden of disease

CU has significant negative impact on quality of life due to its debilitating symptoms [19, 20]. In addition to classic symptoms, like pruritus and wheals, other factors can be equally relevant to the patient, such as the unpredictability of flares, sleep disorders, fatigue, drug related side effects and physical appearance [21]. A major impairment is observed in patients with the highest disease activity and in patients with autoimmune urticaria [21]. Undertreated patients report high disease burden that leads to higher economic burden due to absence or presenteeism - reduced capacity while - at work and higher utilisation of health care resources [19, 20]. Itching and angioedema are the main reasons affecting capacity at work causing presenteeism [22].

Other reasons that contribute to high socio-economic burden include an often considerable delay in diagnosis and specialist referral [22], the inadequate knowledge about CSU in primary and secondary care, and high cost for unnecessary investigations and treatments due to poor adherence to guidelines and best practice [22].

6. Treatment of chronic urticaria

The aim of CU therapy is symptom control as no cure is available to date. Often management of CSU and CINDU overlap. Approach to CU management [2, 10, 19] consists of:

1. Identification and elimination or treatment of underlying causes and associated conditions

2. Avoidance of any known aggravating trigger factors including NSAIDs, ACE-Inhibitors, physical stimuli where possible

3. Pharmacological therapy to prevent MCs degranulation of mediators and their effects [2]

Investigations to rule out any underlying inflammatory or infectious diseases should be initiated on a case-by-case basis. Plasmapheresis has been shown to provide temporary improvement in some autoantibody positive patients with refractory CSU [2] by reducing functional autoantibodies.

Two major professional bodies have published guidelines [1, 19] for the evaluation and management of urticaria. The US JTF Practice Parameter recommends a 4-step approach to management (**Table 7**), whereas the EAACI guidelines (**Table 8**) advocate a 3-step approach. Both guidelines concur in that first line therapy for acute and chronic urticaria should focus on the use of non-sedating 2nd generation H1 antihistamines (SGAs).

The European guidelines differ from the US guidelines in that treatment with sedating 1st generation H1 antihistamines (FGAs) and H2 antihistamines are not recommended. In addition, European guidelines regulate Leukotriene Modifying Agents (LTMAs) to the last Step 3 treatment, whereas US guidelines recommend these agents to be used earlier as adjunctive Step 2 [1].

Although both the US and the European urticaria guidelines recommend a step-by-step approach to CU therapy, patient specific parameters such as serologic, clinical or histological findings are not considered. To date no clinically effective treatment algorithm exists for CU that is based on patient specific parameters [19].

Finally, both the US and European urticaria treatment guidelines should be used with caution and might require adaptation in children, pregnant/lactating women, and elderly patients with CU, as drug doses may have to be reduced or might be contraindicated [1, 2, 19].

US urticaria guidelines to therapy approach
• Begin therapy at the step that is appropriate for individual patient considering urticaria severity and previous treatment history • Medication should be assessed at each step for efficacy and adverse effects • Once adequate control has been achieved it is appropriate to step down treatment
Step 1 • Start Monotherapy with non-sedating 2nd generation antihistamine (SGA) • Avoid any trigger factors (NSAIDs, ACE-Inhibitors) and relevant physical stimuli
Step 2 One or more of the following can be used simultaneously: • Increase up to fourfold the dose of SGA used in Step 1 • Add another SGA • Add a H2-antagonist • Add leukotriene receptor antagonist • Add 1st generation antihistamine (FGA) to be taken at bedtime
Step 3 Advance dose of FGA (hydroxyzine or doxepin) as tolerated
Step 4 Alternative treatment can be added: • Omalizumab or cyclosporine • Other anti-inflammatory agents, immunosuppressants, biologic therapy

Table 7.
Adapted from JTF practice parameters "The diagnosis and management of acute and chronic urticaria: 2014 update" [1].

EAACI Urticaria guidelines to treatment approach

First Line

Monotherapy with 2nd generation antihistamines

↓ If no improvement after 2 weeks

Second Line

Increase dose up to fourfold of 2nd generation antihistamine used as first line

↓ If symptoms persist after another 1- 3 weeks

Third Line

Add one of the following second line agents:
- Omalizumab
- Cyclosporine
- Montelukast

Short course of oral corticosteroids (up to 10 days) can be used at all times during a severe flare

Table 8.
Adapted from EAACI urticaria guideline for the definition, classification, diagnosis and management of urticaria: 2013 revision [1].

6.1 H1-antihistamines

There is good evidence for the use of second-generation antihistamines (SGAs) as first line therapy in mild to moderate CU [1, 7, 19]. SGAs like cetirizine, levocetirizine, loratadine, desloratadine fexofenadine, azelastine, bilastine have a good safety, efficacy and tolerability profile. Over 50% of CU do not respond to the licenced dose of SGAs. For these patients 2–4 times higher than licenced dose is well tolerated and considered acceptable [1, 2, 10, 19]. First generation antihistamines (FGAs) are effective but due to their sedating effect and possible interference with daily activities they are not preferred choice. Side effects include excessive dryness, constipation (due to anticholinergic activity) and occasional Torsades de Pointe (especially linked to astemizole and terfenadine). About 30% of patients continue to experience CU symptoms despite maximal tolerated doses of SGAs [1, 2, 10, 19, 23] and are classified as non-responders [23].

6.2 H2-antihistamines

H2- Antihistamines can be added to H1-antihistamine monotherapy if they prove ineffective. Cimetidine has been shown to increase the half-life of H1-antihistamines [19]. Ranitidine was shown in a Cochrane review to be more effective in combination with diphenhydramine than diphenhydramine on its own [19]. The opinion about their use in combination with H1-antihistamines in the treatment of CU is however divided and is reflected in the difference of recommendation between the US and European urticaria guidelines (**Table 7** vs. **Table 8**). Doxepin a tricyclic antidepressant has combined H1 and H2 and muscarinic blocking activities. It has been shown to be effective in as high as 43% of patients who are recalcitrant to high dose antihistamines therapy [10, 23]. It can be given in doses of 25–50 mg at night or 10-25 mg 3–4 times per day.

6.3 Leukotriene modifier agents (LMAs)

LMAs are leukotriene receptor antagonists and include montelukast and zafirlukast as well as the 5-lipoxygenase-inhibitor zileuton. Several RCTs on CU therapy showed mixed results and thus firm recommendations are not available. However, due the good safety profile of LMAs they might be considered an alternative addition in CU patients who are refractory to antihistamines therapy [17, 24] (**Table 7**). Predictors of good response to LMAs include urticaria triggered by Aspirin, NSAIDs, food additives or pseudoallergens and autoimmune urticaria with positive autologous serum skin prick test [1, 10, 19, 25]. Montelukast can be used in doses of 10 mg/day [10].

6.4 Oral corticosteroids (OCTs)

Large control studies are not available on the use of OCTs in CU. However, OCTs show high efficacy in recalcitrant CU and are used for short term and at the lowest effective dose for severe flares. Long term use of OCTs in CU is not recommended due the multitude of known significant adverse effects [1, 2, 10, 23]. Tapering of OCTs dose is not needed if the patients take <40 mg daily dose and for a period of up to 3 weeks [19]. Oral mini pulses with methyl prednisolone 16 mg tablets twice weekly for 2 months and in combination with H1-antihistamines showed significant reduction in mean UAS7 in a small number of patients [10].

6.5 Immunosuppressive agents (IAs)

IAs should be considered in the case of OCTs therapy being required for longer periods of time. Ciclosporin is the most studied medication and is recommended to be used either at a weight-based dose of 4 mg/kg/per day or at a daily dose of 200 mg for a period of 16 weeks [1, 2, 10, 19]. Improvement in UAS can be as early as 2 weeks of commencing treatment and complete remission occurs in 3 out of 4 patients [10] particularly in autoimmune associated CSU. Regular monitoring is required due to the risk of significant adverse effects and it is reserved in the treatment of severe refractory CSU. Other IAs include:

- Methotrexate
- Mycophenolate Mofetil
- Azathioprine
- Mizoribine
- Intravenous or oral Cyclophosphamide

6.6 Alternative agents

Alternative Agents have also been anecdotally used in refractory CSU and may be of value to individual patients and in certain clinical circumstances [1, 2, 5, 24]. These agents include:

- Dapsone
- Sulfasalazine
- Hydroxychloroquine
- Colchicine
- Intravenous Immunoglobulins
- Plasmapheresis

6.7 NB-UVB therapy

NB-UVB Therapy has been shown in combination with levocetirizine to significantly reduce urticaria activity and to have a long-lasting positive effect on UAS7 [10, 19]. PUVA and BB-UVB have so far shown mixed to neutral results [19].

6.8 Biologic agents

Omalizumab is licenced for the treatment of CU in adults and adolescents that continue to be symptomatic despite the use H1 antihistamines therapy.

Omalizumab is a recombinant humanised IgG monoclonal antibody against the Fc portion of the IgE antibody. It prevents free IgE binding to the high affinity IgE receptor FcεRI and downregulates these receptors on MC and basophils [4, 19]. It has been shown to be effective and well tolerated in 3 phase III and 2 phase II studies at doses from 150 to 300 mg every 4 weeks independent of total serum IgE level or body weight [2, 19]. Omalizumab improves angioedema and quality of life, is suitable for long-term use, and treats relapse after discontinuation [2]. 35–40% of patients achieve complete relief and another 30% reported partial relief after 3 and 6 months [2, 4]. The recommended dose is 300 mg by subcutaneous injection every 4 weeks. Some patients may achieve symptom control with a dose of 150 mg subcutaneous injection every 4 weeks [2]. If no therapeutic response is seen within 6 months of treatment efficacy is unlikely to be achieved and omalizumab can be discontinued [19]. Patients with type I autoimmune CSU experience faster response to omalizumab than type IIb autoimmune CSU. A large real-world US study [26] showed majority of CSU patients started on 300 mg omalizumab dose, were continuously treated for >6 months and without up or down titration for an average of 9 months. 25% of patients that discontinued therapy restarted it. The use of other CU related treatments particularly OCTs was lower after omalizumab commencement [26].

6.9 CSU therapy in special patient groups

The management of CSU in pregnant/lactating women, children and the elderly is largely the same as for non-pregnant adults.

In **pregnant and lactating women** antihistamines should be used at the lowest effective dose [10, 19]. and for the shortest periods of time. SGAs are classified pregnancy category B by US FDA [10]. All antihistamines are secreted in breast milk and use of FGAs is discouraged during lactation to avoid excessive sedation of the breastfed child [10].

A short course of OCTs may be considered during pregnancy, in case of severe exacerbation. Potential side effects include malformation, neonatal adrenal insufficiency, low birth weight. Although OCTs are secreted in breast milk they are generally considered safe during lactation [10].

Omalizumab is classified pregnancy category B by US FDA [10].

In **children** SGAs rather than FGAs should be used as first line therapy and adjusted for age and weight [10, 19].

OCTs should be avoided where possible and if required only used for 10–14 days because of growth related side effects [10, 19]. The use of omalizumab in adolescents is well supported by the current literature and recommended as step 3 and before the use of ciclosporin in the 2017 urticaria guidelines of EAACI/GA^{2}LEN/EDF/WAO [27].

Ciclosporin is recommended as step 4 and was reported effective in a single open label trial of 7 children aged 9–16 years, at the dose of 3 mg/kg/day in two divided doses for maximum of 8 weeks. Regular monitoring of blood pressure and renal function [10] is required.

There is limited data available regarding the up dosing of SGAs and omalizumab in children with CSU under 12 years of age, and the treatment with cyclosporine and LMAs in paediatric patients of all ages [27].

Therapy of CSU in the **elderly** needs to consider comorbidities, polypharmacotherapy and organ insufficiency and adjusted accordingly [19].

7. Conclusions

In summary CSU is a debilitating disease with a relapsing course. It affects 0.5–1% of the population at any given time. The duration of CSU is generally 1–5 years but can be longer in cases associated with angioedema and autoreactivity. CSU has detrimental effects on quality of life with sleep-deprivation and psychiatric disorders being the most frequent.

In a great number of patients an underlying cause or eliciting factor cannot be identified. Among the patients in which an aetiology is suspected, infections, medication, food and psychological factors are most commonly associated. A potential autoimmune cause has been reported in up to 50% of patients. Urticaria can be presenting sign for many syndromes and associated with several conditions. CINDU is characterised by its ability to be triggered consistently and reproducibly in response to a specific stimulus (pressure, temperature, vibration, water, heat, light).

The diagnosis of CU is often made on clinical grounds, a limited routine diagnostic work-up is recommended in a case-by-case basis.

Antihistamines form the mainstay of therapy. In non-responders a variety of other drugs are available including leukotriene receptor inhibitors, conventional systemic therapy, anti-inflammatory and biologic therapy. Special care must be taken when treating children, pregnant/lactating women and the elderly.

Author details

Evmorfia Ladoyanni
Department of Dermatology, University Hospitals Birmingham, Solihull Hospital, Birmingham, United Kingdom

*Address all correspondence to: effil@doctors.org.uk

References

[1] https://www.ncbi.nlm.nih.gov/pmc/articles/PMC4921693/

[2] https://dermnetnz.org/topics/chronic-spontaneous-urticaria/

[3] https://www.ncbi.nlm.nih.gov/pmc/articles/PMC5625775/

[4] https://www.ncbi.nlm.nih.gov/pmc/articles/PMC6450064/

[5] C Antia, K Baquerizo, A Korman et al. Urticaria: A comprehensive review, J Am Acad Dermatol. 2018;79:599-614

[6] https://www.ncbi.nlm.nih.gov/pmc/articles/PMC4756797/

[7] https://www.ncbi.nlm.nih.gov/pmc/articles/PMC7661155/

[8] https://www.ncbi.nlm.nih.gov/pmc/articles/PMC6737621/

[9] https://www.ncbi.nlm.nih.gov/pmc/articles/PMC7265766/

[10] https://www.ncbi.nlm.nih.gov/pmc/articles/PMC4458932/

[11] https://www.ncbi.nlm.nih.gov/pmc/articles/PMC5506533/

[12] CY Chu, YT Cho, JH Jiang et al. Patients with chronic urticaria have a higher risk of psychiatric disorders: a population based study, Br J Dermatol. 2020: 182:335-341

[13] https://www.ncbi.nlm.nih.gov/pmc/articles/PMC4713874/

[14] https://www.ncbi.nlm.nih.gov/pmc/articles/PMC6936629/

[15] https://www.ncbi.nlm.nih.gov/pmc/articles/PMC4985525/

[16] https://www.ncbi.nlm.nih.gov/pmc/articles/PMC6760047/

[17] https://www.ncbi.nlm.nih.gov/pmc/articles/PMC7170265/

[18] https://www.ncbi.nlm.nih.gov/pmc/articles/PMC5978890/

[19] C Antia, K Baquerizo, A Korman et al. Urticaria: A comprehensive review, J Am Acad Dermatol. 2018;79:617-633

[20] https://www.ncbi.nlm.nih.gov/pmc/articles/PMC7726718/

[21] https://www.ncbi.nlm.nih.gov/pmc/articles/PMC5193185/

[22] https://www.ncbi.nlm.nih.gov/pmc/articles/PMC5724512/

[23] https://www.ncbi.nlm.nih.gov/pmc/articles/PMC5515622/

[24] https://www.ncbi.nlm.nih.gov/pmc/articles/PMC6439569/

[25] https://www.ncbi.nlm.nih.gov/pmc/articles/PMC3048602/

[26] https://www.ncbi.nlm.nih.gov/pmc/articles/PMC5911510/

[27] https://www.ncbi.nlm.nih.gov/pmc/articles/PMC7955742/

Chapter 3

Clinical Phenotypes in NSAID-Induced Urticaria/Angioedema

Joaquin Quiralte, María del Robledo Ávila, Stefan Cimbollek and Joaquin Quiralte-Castillo

Abstract

The skin clinical phenotypes of nonsteroidal anti-inflammatory drug (NSAID) hypersensitivity (NH) are very heterogeneous with several syndromes after NSAID intake, which include different symptoms, different organ involvement and different associated concomitant diseases and possibly different underlying pathophysiology and mechanisms. Making a correct diagnosis in NH is an exciting journey for any allergist. Thus, to classify these diseases properly will be pivotal for appropriate diagnostic and management strategy. Treatment modalities are depending on the clinical phenotypes of NH and they will embrace for each patient: the avoidance of culprit NSAID, the finding of well-tolerated NSAID and in certain cases, desensitization procedures when the NSAID treatment was absolutely needed as well as the control of associated diseases such as spontaneous chronic urticarial or allergic respiratory diseases. This review updates the recent evidence of classification, diagnostic strategies, and management of skin NSAID hypersensitivity reactions.

Keywords: NSAID hypersensitivity, urticaria, angioedema, single-blind placebo-controlled oral challenge, management

1. Introduction

Nonsteroidal anti-inflammatory drugs (NSAID) are one of the most commonly used drugs worldwide. NSAIDs are a major cause of hypersensitivity reactions, and they suppose up to half the cases of adverse reactions evaluated in a tertiary allergy unit [1]. Adverse reactions to NSAIDs account for 12% to 29.6% of all adverse reactions in hospital admissions. Most adverse reactions to NSAIDs belong to type A, which are dose-dependent and predictable from their pharmacological actions. Common type A reactions include gastrointestinal bleeding and acute kidney injury. Type B reactions, also known as NSAID hypersensitivity (NH) reactions, account for 8.4% to 18.3% of total adverse reactions to NSAID [2]. NSAIDs are a large and chemically heterogeneous group of drugs that inhibit the enzyme cyclooxygenase (COX) 1 and 2 isoforms, an so block the production of prostaglandins from arachidonic acid.

NSAIDs are typically divided into groups based on their chemical structure and selectivity for blocking COX-2: acetylated salicylates (aspirin), non-acetylated salicylates (diflunisal, salsalate), propionic acids (naproxen, ibuprofen, dexketoprofen), acetic acids (diclofenac, indomethacin, aceclofenac, tolmetin), enolic acids (meloxicam, piroxicam), anthranilic acids (meclofenamate, mefenamic acid, niflumic acid), naphthylalanine (nabumetone), pyrazolones (metamizole, propyfenazone) and selective COX-2 inhibitors (celecoxib, etoricoxib).

Several distinct clinical syndromes are described regarding NH, most often manifested as respiratory reactions (e.g, bronchospasm and nasoocular reaction), urticaria/angioedema or systemic anaphylaxis. NH often appears in patients who also suffer certain concomitant diseases, such as chronic rhinosinusitis with nasal polyps and bronchial asthma or spontaneous chronic urticaria. Both, the type of reaction after NSAID exposure and the concomitant associated disease are critical to classify the NH [3]. The focus of this chapter will provide an overview on all the aspects of skin NSAID hypersensitivity immediate reactions, from clinical symptoms to leading practical recommendations with respect to diagnosis and management.

2. A working classification of skin NSAID hypersensitivity based on clinical phenotypes

Controlled oral challenge is the only definitive way to diagnose the reactions caused by NSAIDs. These challenge-proven immediate responses are a wide group of disorders that includes respiratory, cutaneous and anaphylaxis reactions [1, 3].

The mechanisms of NH are unknown, but two general hypotheses have been proposed [4]. The first one, an enzymatic activity inhibition of at least the cyclooxygenase-1 (COX-1) isoform that may inhibit the prostaglandin synthesis and thus deregulate the 5-lipooxygenase pathway, with cys-leukotriene hyperproduction in some susceptible patients. All NSAIDs that inhibit the COX-1 isoform could precipitate the reaction. For this reason, cross-reactivity among COX-1 inhibitor NSAIDs can be demonstrated in all patients with respiratory reactions and in most patients with urticaria/angioedema reactions (multiple reactors) [1, 3, 4]. The second mechanism can be applied only to a small subset of patients with NSAID hypersensitivity, as those with systemic anaphylaxis [4]. We have previously demonstrated that patients with NSAIDs-induced systemic anaphylaxis can react only to one specific NSAIDs and tolerate other COX-1 inhibitor NSAIDs in controlled oral challenges. Up to 1/3 of patients with NSAID induced systemic anaphylaxis might present immediate acute urticarial previous to anaphylactic episode when taken a specific NSAID (selective reactors) [3–5].

At least, three subsets of these patients with NH may have an associated underlying disease: in fact, around 10 percent of patients with chronic rhinosinusitis with nasal polyps and moderate-to-severe asthma and 30 percent of those with chronic urticaria/angioedema may present a nasoocular/asthmatic or urticarial reaction after NSAID exposure at some times in their lives, respectively [6]. Some clinical phenotypes of skin NSAID hypersensitivity are also definitely associated with allergic respiratory disease [3, 7].

Therefore, the diagnostic approach determines very different clusters of patients [3, 8]. Those who present clinical reactivity between different NSAIDs (multiple reactors) versus those who develop a reaction exclusively to a specific NSAID (selective reactors), and secondly, those in whom there is a very defined concomitant associated disease from the clinical and biological point of view. NSAID exposure exacerbates these diseases, determining a clinical reaction. However, the NSAID withdrawal does not determine a notable modification of the natural history of the disease, which often must continue to be treated despite the avoidance of NSAID [8].

Therefore, the NSAID reaction is an epiphenomenon that together with other clinical features constitutes what we have called the clinical phenotype (formerly called the NSAID-reaction complex) [1, 3]. This classification based on clinical phenotypes is a real and practical approach in the daily clinic, which will allow us to make the best appropriate diagnostic and therapeutic decisions.

3. The skin clinical phenotypes of NSAID hypersensitivity

The skin reactions are the most prevalent clinical phenotypes in patients with NSAID hypersensitivity. We have described at least 5 clinical phenotypes of immediate-type of skin NSAID hypersensitivity: [3, 7] NSAID-exacerbated cutaneous disease (NECD), NSAID-induced urticaria/angioedema (NIUA), two clinical phenotypes (NSAID induced isolated periorbital angioedema and NSAID induced recall urticarial) which are present exclusively in patients with respiratory allergy, mainly house dust mites; and a single NSAID induced urticaria/angioedema/anaphylaxis (SNIUAA) (**Table 1**). The last mentioned is probably an IgE-mediated allergy. The remaining phenotypes do not have an immunological pathophysiology, but are caused by inhibiting COX-1 resulting in an imbalance in eicosanoid mediators, as above outlined.

3.1 The NSAID-exacerbated cutaneous disease

Patients with NECD suffer from spontaneous chronic urticaria and/or angioedema (CSU) and experience a worsening of these symptoms after NSAID intake. Most reactions appear between 1 to 12 hours after administering NSAID and last several days until the reaction is controlled with supplemental doses of antihistamines and/or corticosteroids. In up to 30 percent of cases facial, neck and hand angioedema may occur during the clinical exacerbation; an isolated angioedema is rarely a possible manifestation of NECD. Approximately 30% of patients with chronic spontaneous urticaria present exacerbations of their disease after NSAID exposure throughout their lives [1, 3–5, 8]. A positive correlation between the basal CSU activity disease and the possibility of a NSAID challenge reaction have been described in NECD patients [8].

NSAID reactivity pattern	Clinical form	Associated underlying diseases
Cross-reactive syndromes	NSAID-exacerbated cutaneous disease	Spontaneous chronic urticaria/angioedema
	NSAID-induced urticarial/ angioedema	
	NSAID-induced isolated periorbital angioedema	Allergic respiratory diseases
		Oral mite anaphylaxis
	NSAID- induced recall urticaria	Allergic respiratory diseases treated with subcutaneous allergen immunotherapy
Selective syndromes	Urticaria/systemic anaphylaxis	

Table 1.
Skin clinical phenotypes of NSAID hypersensitivity.

Since CSU is often a self-limiting disease within months to years, NECD can potentially remit with the resolution of CSU. However, NECD patients seem to have a distinct phenotype compared with NSAID-tolerant CSU patients: the latter have a shorter duration of CSU and less often have angioedema when compared with NECD patients [9].

3.2 NSAID-induced urticaria/angioedema

Patients with NSAID-induced urticaria and/or angioedema (NIUA) do not have spontaneous urticaria and/or angioedema, but only the reactions develop after the NSAID intake. NIUA is a multiple NSAID hypersensitivity syndrome and there is cross-reactivity between chemically unrelated NSAIDs. Since patients often start to avoid NSAIDs after their first reaction, this cross-reactivity might not always be clear. Patients can report isolated urticaria, angioedema or a combination of both. A small proportion of patients with NIUA developed chronic spontaneous urticaria after 10 year- period of follow-up [10]. So, there is a certain degree of interrelationship between both phenotypes, NECD and NIUA, and possibly in some patients they represent different stages of the same disease.

All patients with NECD and NIUA show a pattern of multiple reactivity between NSAID, dependent on the level of *in vitro* inhibition potency of COX −1 isoform (**Table 2**).

3.3 Isolated periorbital angioedema (iPA), or the infanto-juvenile form of NH

This type of reaction usually affects children and young people, with an onset in the first or second decade of life in more than 80% of cases and, in all cases, an associated respiratory allergy is detected, mostly caused by mites, suggesting a close relationship with aspirin exacerbated respiratory disease (AERD) with which they share not only the concomitant disease, but also the pattern of multiple reactivity among NSAID [3, 6].

Category	Drug	Doses
Placebo	Lactose	
Highly selective COX-2 inhibitor	Celecoxib	50, 100, 200 [a]
	Etoricoxib	30, 60 [a]
Preferential COX-2 inhibitor	Meloxicam	7.5, 15 mg [a]
Weak, non-discriminatory COX-1/COX-2 inhibitor	Paracetamol	100, 250, 500, 1000 mg [a]
Potent, non-discriminatory COX-1/COX-2 inhibitor	Diclofenac	25, 50 mg [b]
	Ibuprofen	50, 150, 250, 600 mg [a, d]
	Metamizole	10, 50, 125, 250, 575 mg [a, e]
	Acetylsalycilic acid	50, 100, 250, 500 mg [c, f]

Drugs were administered in an opaque capsule at the following intervals between each dose: [a]60 minutes, [b]120 minutes and [c]180 minutes. [d]Three doses, [e]four doses or [f]two doses were administered on the first day, and [d, e]one dose or [f]two other doses on the second day.

Table 2.
NSAIDs and doses used for single-blind, placebo controlled oral challenge.

Within this group of patients and in close relationship with the atopic phenomenon, a new syndrome has been described: the systemic anaphylaxis triggered by ingestion of food contaminated by mites (NSAIDs sensitivity mite-ingestion reaction syndrome or also recently called oral mite anaphylaxis) [11, 12]. Most of the patients presented common clinical characteristics: they had respiratory allergy to mites, presented mostly periorbital angioedema and presented anaphylactic episodes of variable severity in relation to the ingestion of food made with cereal flour (wheat, oat and corn), without any evidence of food allergy during the clinical study. 87% of the study group presented intolerance to aspirin, contrasting with the frequency of less than 2% that we observed in the population of patients allergic to domestic dust mites. This meant that an atopic aspirin intolerant was up to 300 times more likely to suffer a severe reaction from ingestion of mites than a tolerant patient. Microscopic analysis of the flour revealed extreme contamination of the flour by *Dermatophagoides farinae* and other mites of the Acaridae family (specifically *Tyreophagus entomophagus* and *Suidasia medinensis*). At present, the cause of the association of aspirin intolerance with systemic reactions by ingestion of food contaminated by mites is unknown.

3.4 NSAID-induced recall urticaria

Recall urticaria (RU) is a rare biologic phenomenon characterized by the existence of hives only in the previously injected site when the patient is exposed again from another source. The most common example are patients who have received previously subcutaneous allergen immunotherapy (sq AIT) and present focal skin reaction at the sites of previous allergens injection when a new kind of allergen shot was administered or after heavy ambiental exposure to the allergen [13].

We recently described a patient with allergic respiratory disease who underwent sq. AIT to house dust mites after a 5 year-period. Two years after allergen immunotherapy discontinuation, patient first experienced an immediate local urticarial reaction with multiple hives at previous sq. AIT injection sites after metamizole and ibuprofen intake. SBPCOC with ibuprofen and aspirin was performed and elicited multiples hives in a circumscribed area in both arms, although a controlled challenge with celecoxib was negative.

In our patient, the symptoms were elicited by different NSAIDs (Ibuprofen, metamizol and aspirin) which resembles the pattern of patients with skin cross-reactive phenotypes of NSAID hypersensitivity. This suggests that the enzymatic inhibition of COX type I isoform could play a role in the development of this specific reaction. The tolerance of highly selective COX type 2 inhibitors such as celecoxib in our patient reinforces this hypothesis. However, the nature of the relationship between COX-1 inhibition and the local immunological trace of mite remains largely unknown. This phenomenon might be a new phenotype of skin NSAID hypersensitivity which would appear in those patients with respiratory allergy treated with sq. AIT [7].

3.5 Selective acute urticaria/angioedema and anaphylaxis

The existence of underlying diseases is common in NECD, NIUA and IPA. However, there is another phenotype of otherwise healthy patients, (i.e. without any concomitant disease associated) who experience immediate reactions of urticarial or anaphylactic type after the administration of a specific NSAID [1, 3–5, 8].

Up to 15% of patients with NSAID-induced urticaria present a selective pattern of sensitivity to NSAIDs, [8] with a predominance of certain NSAID groups, such as those derived from the pyrazole group (metamizole) followed in order of frequency by ibuprofen, diclofenac and paracetamol, A selective pattern involves SBPCOC tolerance to other NSAIDs not involved in the clinical reaction, including those that are potent inhibitors of COX isoform 1.

Immediate systemic reactions present clinical and biological features that are compatible with a possible immunological mechanism: they are generally anaphylactic, selective and, on certain occasions, can be associated with positive skin tests that can be read immediately (such as metamizole) [14].

Recently, Doña et el have described some patients who may develop immediate reactions to several NSAIDs but tolerate ASA (the NSAIDs-multiple selective immediate reaction phenotype). Patients usually present with a biselective or triselective pattern: they presented different episodes of anaphylaxis to ibuprofen and diclofenac while tolerate an aspirin challenge or developing hypersensitivity reactions to three non chemically related NSAIDs [1].

Although the selective form is the most frequent clinical form of NSAID anaphylaxis (96%), a small subgroup of patients with phenotypes associated with multiple reactivity can present an anaphylactic reaction during SBPCOC. Patients with NIUA and exceptionally periorbital angioedema may present with a systemic reaction after administration of a potent COX-1 inhibitor NSAID. In rare cases, the systemic reaction may be a clinical phenotype in itself, with patients exhibiting this clinical response to any exposure to NSAID [3].

4. Diagnostic strategy in skin reactions to NSAID

The main tools that allow us to deal with cutaneous reactions to NSAIDs are the clinical history and controlled re-exposure to NSAIDs in a hospital setting [3]. The careful and complete review of clinical reactions to NSAID is essential before any challenge procedure and allows us to provisionally classify the patient with NH, while the latter, the SBPCOC, definitively assigns the patient to a specific phenotype. Our objective is to offer the best analgesic, anti-inflammatory or antiplatelet alternatives in the event that the patient tolerates the NSAID without reaction.

4.1 To classify, to classify, to classify...always

The clinical history is the basic method of temporarily assigning the patient to a specific clinical phenotype. The phenotypic classification of any patient with a possible NH (**Table 1**) will be the first (and the most important) diagnostic step in the investigation of these types of reactions. Properly classifying NH will help us to choose safest diagnostic approach for each patient [1, 3–5, 8].

The first key element to classify these patients will be the time elapsed between the administration of NSAID and the beginning of the reaction. The so-called latency time allow us to differentiate the reactions in: immediate (less than 24 hours, usually between 1 and 2 hours) and delayed reactions (over 24 hours). Secondly, we will have to evaluate the clinical manifestations of the reaction (respiratory, cutaneous or systemic), the NSAID involved, the route of administration and the reason why the drug was prescribed, as well as the coexistence of associated concomitant diseases (chronic rhinosinusitis with nasosinusal polyposis, bronchial asthma, spontaneous chronic urticaria or allergic respiratory disease). Thirdly, we will have to determine the NSAID tolerated previously and after the reaction. This will allow us to make a first historical approach to NSAID reactivity status: multiple reactor with reactivity among non-chemically related NSAIDs (**Table 3**) or selective reactor with sensitivity to a single NSAID with tolerance to at least one potent COX-1 inhibitor NSAID (**Table 4**).

Therefore, the classification of patients based on clinical phenotypes is critical in addressing diagnostic and therapeutic strategies in these patients. The identification of comorbidities such as chronic spontaneous urticaria, allergic respiratory disease or reactions to mite-contaminated cereal flour-based foods are key clinical elements that might define a phenotype and predict in most cases multiple reactivity to different groups of NSAIDs. The worsening of spontaneous chronic urticaria after NSAID administration and the development of the reaction within 1 to 6 hours of NSAID administration are common clinical features that can be referred up in most patients with skin-type reactions.

In a percentage of cases, clinical information on reactivity status is limited, either because the patient has had only a single reaction with a single NSAID or because of the impossibility of determining each of the NSAIDs involved in the patient's lifetime reactions. In these cases, determining this status is essential to approach a therapeutic plan. The only way to determine the reactivity status is through SBPCDC with NSAIDs that have differential inhibition against each of isoforms COX-1 and COX-2. However, we could collect in the clinical history some findings that may allow us to identify a multiple or selective reactor status (**Tables 3** and **4**). In general, a NSAID highly selective for COX-2 inhibition, such as a COXIb, will be better tolerated than a potent COX 1–2 inhibitor in patients who are multiple reactors. The degree of COX inhibition is directly proportional to the probability of reaction and the intensity of its clinical manifestations [1, 3–5, 8]. In the case of a selective reactor, all COX-1 inhibitor NSAIDs will be tolerated, except the one involved in the historical reaction (or those which are chemically related).

• Urticaria/angioedema which appear between 1 to 6 hours to NSAID intake
• Bilateral periorbital angioedema after NSAID intake in children
• Nasoocular and/or asthmatic reaction after NSAID intake
• Historical reactions to other non-chemically related NSAID
• Chronic rhinosinusitis with nasal polyps
• Moderate-to-severe bronchial asthma
• Spontaneous chronic urticaria
• Inducible (dermographism, cholinergic) chronic urticaria
• Allergic respiratory disease to house dust mites
• Systemic reaction after flour-based food ingestion

Table 3.
Clinical findings suggesting a NSAID multiple reactor.

• Urticaria which appear within 1 h to NSAID intake
• Inmediate Systemic anaphylaxis after NSAID administration
• Historical tolerance to other non-chemically potent COX-1 inhibitor NSAID
• No concomitant associated diseases

Table 4.
Clinical findings suggesting a selective reactor status.

4.2 Principles to design the best controlled oral challenge for each clinical phenotype

The fundamental objectives of SBPCOC is threefold: **first**, to determine the clinical syndrome associated with the reaction after administration of the NSAID. In the case of systemic anaphylaxis due to an NSAID, the use of the NSAID involved during the clinical reaction is completely contraindicated. **Second**, determine the tolerance pattern to NSAIDs in an individual patient. A negative SBPCOC will determine the NSAID reintroduction of the treatment in the patient with NH. The stratification of NSAID according to their inhibitory potency of each of the COX1 and COX2 isoenzymes determines the likelihood of reaction and therefore the order of administration of NSAIDs during SBPCOC [15]. Thus, for example, in a patient with diclofenac and ibuprofen-induced NIUA, a SBPCOC with celecoxib or etoricoxib is highly likely to be tolerated (and therefore included in the self-care plan for patient management) while an SBPCOC with another strong COX-1 inhibitor NSAID is highly likely to induce a reaction, diagnose the patient, and determine a multiple pattern of reactivity. And **third** and finally, it allows us to initiate a desensitization procedure in patients with immediate respiratory or cutaneous reactions requiring a desensitization procedure that determines the introduction of an NSAID for anti-inflammatory or antiaggregant treatment if necessary. Desensitization is a procedure which will be discussed later and which determines a temporary state of tolerance while the administration of the NSAID persists.

4.2.1 SBPCOC with NSAID in patients with cross-reactive skin reactions

The approach to patients with the various phenotypes of cross-reactive skin reactions (NECD, NIUA, IPA and NIRU) is very similar. We always have to bear in mind that these patients seek our advice because they lack analgesic and anti-inflammatory alternative strategy, and their fundamental objective is to find an alternative that will solve their underlying disease without inducing a reaction. Therefore, the stratification of SBPCOC with NSAIDs plays an essential role in these cases, since it is directly related to a potential positive response during the challenge [15]. In virtually all cases these patients tolerate COXiB. Even in the rare cases where they do not tolerate a given COXiB, it is essential to expose them to another COXiB as it can be otherwise tolerated [16].

NSAIDs, which are COX2 inhibitors, but which inhibit COX-1 in a dose-dependent manner, such as meloxicam, would be the next alternative to propose in these patients. Paracetamol, a weak COX-1 and COX-2 inhibitor, is generally tolerated at the time of the clinical history by most patients. Its analgesic potential, but the absence of anti-inflammatory effects, is what finally decides the patient to go to the allergist looking for more appropriate alternatives. The use of potent COX1 and COX2 inhibitors, such as aspirin, ibuprofen, metamizole or diclofenac necessarily determine a reaction and therefore a diagnosis in this type of reaction [3, 8, 15].

4.2.2 SBPCOC with NSAID in patients with selective urticaria and anaphylaxis

The existence of an NSAID-induced anaphylaxis predicts the existence of a selective pattern that in many cases can already be detected in the clinical history, because the patient has tolerance to other non-chemically related NSAIDs. In a study of patients with NSAID anaphylaxis we have demonstrated that patients tolerated with impunity any NSAID, if we avoided the historically implicated NSAID or other chemically related NSAIDs during the SBPC [3]. In the group of patients with pyrazolone (metamizole, propyfenazone) anaphylaxis in Spain, skin tests (prick test at 400 mg/mL and ID at 4 mg/mL) are extremely useful tools to detect an IgE-mediated allergy to these drugs. A positive metamizole skin test will always determine a safe SBPCDC if another non-pyrazolone NSAID is used during challenge. With other NSAIDs, in my experience, skin tests have extremely low sensitivity.

4.2.3 Treating reactions during SBPCOC

NSAID challenges always pose a certain risk, depending on the phenotype of the patient. Therefore, these challenges should be performed by experienced specialized nurses and allergists with the appropriate resources and access to emergency medical and intensive care.

4.3 The single-blind, placebo controlled oral challenge with NSAID: how do we do it?

The SBPCOC with NSAID is the gold standard for the diagnosis of skin NH. SBPCOC is indicated in 3 main scenarios: 1) to confirm/discard if the NSAID involved in the reaction is responsible (especially in those cases where the history is not very suggestive of a reaction to NSAID); 2) To confirm/exclude multiple reactivity among potent COX-1 inhibitors with another NSAID, usually aspirin; and 3) to identify potential alternative NSAIDs that are well tolerated by the patients.

However, there are several clinical situations in which it is contraindicated: If there is severe or uncontrolled bronchial asthma, active spontaneous urticaria/angioedema, pregnancy, active infection, and a recent vaccination ($\leq$ 1 week) and uncontrolled psychiatric disorders. Relative contraindications are also the use of beta-blockers or ACE-inhibitors.

We propose an order of administration of NSAIDs trying to stratify them according to the in vitro potency of COX-1 and COX-2 inhibition (**Table 2**) [3, 14]. This risk stratification management makes us start with, some of the selective COX-2 inhibitors (etoricoxib and celecoxib). Later, if there is no clinical response, the preferential COX-2 NSAIDs are continued (with a dose-dependent inhibitory effect on COX-1, as was the case with meloxicam). Thirdly, if there is no clinical response, a weak NSAID inhibiting both isoforms (e.g. paracetamol) will be administered; to continue, finally, with the potent COX-1 and COX-2 inhibitors.

Stratification of NSAIDs according to their COX-1 inhibition potency allows, to generate effective alternatives that these patients can take if the response during SBPCOC is negative; and to confirm the pattern of reactivity between NSAIDs that allows us to classify clinical phenotypes appropriately.

In the case of NECD the ideal is to carry out the study in a period of remission of chronic spontaneous urticaria. If this is not possible, we will titrate the treatment with antihistamines until the minimum effective control dose is achieved and then perform the SBPCOC. A complete withdrawal of all anti-histamines may determine a high rate of false positives in this subset of patients with NH [8].

The existence of NSAID anaphylaxis contraindicates the use of that specific NSAID or other structurally related one during SBPCOC [3, 8]. However, this type of reaction presents a selective pattern of sensitivity to NSAID, and even those with high COX-1 inhibition potency can be taken with impunity.

5. The management of skin NSAID hypersensitivity

The management of skin reactions to NSAIDs will aim to educate the patient on which drugs to avoid and to provide written therapeutic advice on which alternatives to NSAIDs are potentially safe, after having tested adequate tolerance to them through SBPCOC.

Depending on the diagnosis and outcome of the SBPCOC, the patient can be advised to avoid only the culprit or all NSAID. Then, there might be a need to investigate the safety of other alternative analgesics. Selective COX-2 inhibitors are often a safe alternative, especially in cross-reactive patients who can tolerate acetaminophen. So, below 5% of patients with skin NH reacted to a selective COX-2 inhibitor [17, 18]. Even in those cases with a COXiB reaction, it is possible that the patient may tolerate other COXib without reaction and therefore an second challenge with an alternative COXIb must be performed [16].

Early presentations of periorbital angioedema as key features of cross-reactive reactions to NSAIDs in an atopic children also precluded the use of potent COX-1 inhibitor NSAID. Paracetamol is often well tolerated in these patients. The use of a cyclooxygenase-2-specific medication may not be feasible in this population, and limits options for other medical antiinflammatory treatment. However, Loh et al. have recently demonstrated that etoricoxib can be used as a safe alternative in older children (mean age 13,5 years) with hypersensitivity to multiple antipyretics [19].

Patient with selective urticaria or systemic anaphylaxis presents a selective pattern of sensitivity to NSAID, and even those with high COX-1 inhibition potency, but non chemically related, can be tolerated [3, 5].

Desensitization with aspirin is recommended by clinical guidelines only in patients with aspirin exacerbated respiratory disease and in cases of NECD or NIUA, in which it is strictly necessary to administer any NSAID as an anti-aggregate, anti-inflammatory or analgesic treatment [20]. The desensitization procedure consists of administering progressively increasing doses of aspirin until a reaction is provoked which is as controllable as possible, with the aim of inducing a post-reaction refractory period and which we will use to reach the therapeutic dose, culminating the desensitization process after the administration of a dose of aspirin (or other NSAID) without a reaction.

Rossini et al. have published a multicenter, prospective study that demonstrates that a rapid standardized desensitization protocol in patients with aspirin hypersensitivity undergoing coronary angiography is safe and effective, irrespective of the type of NH which have the patients. A low-dose aspirin could be safely continued without reaction in all patients throughout the next year [20].

6. Conclusions

We have clinically characterized a large population of patients with skin NSAID-induced reactions by means of controlled oral challenges, and we have proposed a working classification of these clinical entities, which can be recognized through the distinct clinical features and the challenge results. Skin NSAID hypersensitivity have showed at least 5 well-defined clinical phenotypes. This classification based on clinical phenotypes is a real and practical approach in the daily clinic, which will allow us to make the best-appropriated diagnostic and therapeutic decisions.

Conflict of interest

The authors declare no conflict of interest.

Author details

Joaquin Quiralte[1]*, María del Robledo Ávila[1], Stefan Cimbollek[1] and Joaquin Quiralte-Castillo[2]

1 Allergy Unit-Hospital Universitario Virgen del Rocio, Seville, Spain

2 Department of Pediatrics, Hospital Juan Ramón Jiménez, Huelva, Spain

*Address all correspondence to: joaquinquiralte@gmail.com

References

[1] Doña I, Pérez-Sánchez N, Eguiluz-Gracia I, Muñoz-Cano R, Bartra J, José Torres MJ, Cornejo-García JA. Progress in understanding hypersensitivity reactions to nonsteroidal anti-inflammatory drugs. Allergy 2020; 75: 561-575. doi: 10.1111/all.14032.

[2] Walters KM, Woessner KM. An Overview of Nonsteroidal Anti-inflammatory Drug Reactions Immunology and Allergy Clinics of North America 2016; 36: 625-641. doi: 10.1016/j.iac.2016.06.001.

[3] Quiralte J, Blanco C, Delgado J, Ortega N, Alcántara M, Castillo R, Anguita JL, Sáenz de San Pedro B, Carrillo T. Challenge-based clinical patterns of 223 Spanish patients with nonsteroidal anti-inflammatory-drug-induced-reactions.J Investig Allergol Clin Immunol. 2007; 17:182-8.

[4] Yeung WYW, Park HS. Update on the Management of Nonsteroidal Anti-Inflammatory Drug Hypersensitivity. Yonsei Med J 2020; 61: 4-14. doi: 10.3349/ymj.2020.61.1.4

[5] Lee Y, Shin YS, Park HS. New phenotypes in hypersensitivity reactions to nonsteroidal anti-inflammatory drugs. Curr Opin Allergy Clin Immunol 2019; 19: 302-307. doi: 10.1097/ACI.0000000000000541.

[6] Laidlaw TM. Clinical updates in aspirin-exacerbated respiratory disease. Allergy Asthma Proc 2019; 40: 4-6. doi: 10.2500/aap.2019.40.4188.

[7] Cimbollek S, Ávila-Castellano MR, Labella M, Baynova K, Aramburu T, Quiralte J. Recall Urticaria: Aspirin Also Induces It. J Investig Allergol Clin Immunol 2018; 28: 131-132. doi: 10.18176/jiaci.0219.

[8] Kowalski ML, Asero R, Bavbek S, Blanca B, Blanca-Lopez N, Bochenek G, Brockow K, Campo P, Celik G, Cernadas J, Cortellini G, Gomes E, Niżankowska-Mogilnicka E, Romano A, Szczeklik A, Testi S, Torres MJ, Wöhrl S, Makowska J. Classification and practical approach to the diagnosis and management of hypersensitivity to nonsteroidal anti-inflammatory drugs. Allergy 2013; 68: 1219-32. doi: 10.1111/all.12260.

[9] Sanchez-Borges M, Caballero-Fonseca F, Capriles-Hulett A, Gonzalez-Aveledo L. Aspirin-exacerbated cutaneous disease (AECD) is a distinct subphenotype of chronic spontaneous urticaria. J Eur Acad Dermatol Venereol. 2015; 29: 698-701. doi: 10.1111/jdv.12658.

[10] Asero R. Intolerance to nonsteroidal anti-inflammatory drugs might precede by years the onset of chronic urticaria. J Allergy Clin Immunol. 2003; 111:1095-8. doi: 10.1067/mai.2003.1444.

[11] Blanco C, Quiralte J, Castillo R, Delgado J, Arteaga C, Barber D, Carrillo T. Anaphylaxis after ingestion of wheat flour contaminated with mites. J Allergy Clin Immunol 1997; 99: 308-13. doi: 10.1016/s0091-6749(97)70047-2.

[12] Sánchez-Borges M, Capriles-Hulett A, Fernandez-Caldas E. Oral mite anaphylaxis: who, when, and how?. Curr Opin Allergy Clin Immunol 2020; 20: 242-247. doi: 10.1097/ACI.0000000000000624.

[13] Ta V, White AA. An unusual case of recurrent "recall urticaria" in a patient on immunotherapy. .J Allergy Clin Immunol Pract 2014; 2:459-460. doi: 10.1016/j.jaip.2014.03.003.

[14] Blanca-López N, Pérez-Sánchez N, Agúndez JA, García-Martin E, Torres MJ, Cornejo-García JA, Perkins JR, Miranda MA, Andreu I, Mayorga C, Canto G, Blanca M, Doña I. Allergic Reactions to Metamizole: Immediate

and Delayed Responses. Int Arch Allergy Immunol 2016; 169: 223-30. doi: 10.1159/000444798

[15] Quiralte J, Sáenz de San Pedro B, Florido JJ. Safety of selective cyclooxygenase-2 inhibitor rofecoxib in patients with NSAID-induced cutaneous reactions. Ann Allergy Asthma Immunol 2002; 89: 63-6. doi: 10.1016/s1081-1206(10)61912-6.

[16] Cimbollek S, Quiralte J, Avila R. COX-2 inhibitors in patients with sensitivity to nonselective NSAIDs. N Engl J Med 2009; 361): 2197-8. doi: 10.1056/NEJMc0907208.

[17] Hermans MAW, Otten R, Karim AF, van Maaren MS. Nonsteroidal anti-inflammatory drug hypersensitivity: not always an allergy!. Neth J Med. 2018 Mar;76(2):52-59.

[18] Llanora GV, Ling Loo EX, Gerez IF, Cheng YK, Shek LP. Etoricoxib: a safe alternative for NSAID intolerance in Asian patients. Asian Pac J Allergy Immunol 2013; 31: 330-3. doi: 10.12932/AP0290.31.4.2013.

[19] Loh W, Lim HL, Rao R, Goh A, Ong LX, Chiang WC. Tolerance to etoricoxib in children with nonsteroidal anti-inflammatory drug hypersensitivity. Asia Pac Allergy 2015; 5: 40-6. doi: 10.5415/apallergy.2015.5.1.40.

[20] Rossini R, Iorio A, Pozzi R, Bianco M, Musumeci G, Leonardi S, Lettieri C, Bossi I, Colombo P, Rigattieri S, Dossena C, Anzuini A, Capodanno D, Senni M, Angiolillo DJ. Aspirin Desensitization in Patients With Coronary Artery Disease: Results of the Multicenter ADAPTED Registry (Aspirin Desensitization in Patients With Coronary Artery Disease). Circ Cardiovasc Interv 2017; 10: e004368. doi: 10.1161/CIRCINTERVENTIONS.116.004368.

Chapter 4

The Use of Omalizumab in Chronic Urticaria: Available Data and Future Aspects of Anti-IgE Treatment

Young-Min Ye

Abstract

Chronic urticaria (CU) defined as repeatedly occurred itchy wheals and/or angioedema for at least 6 weeks. Due to the unpredictability, recurrent and disabling symptoms, and a considerably impaired quality of life, effective and tolerable treatment for CU patients is crucial. Almost a half of patients with CU are refractory to H1-antihistamines, even though the dose of antihistamines is increased up to 4-fold. Recently treatment modulating IgE levels and activities provides an efficient therapeutic approach. Omalizumab, the only approved anti-IgE treatment for chronic spontaneous urticaria (CSU) patients until now, with a strong evidence of the efficacy and safety, opened a new horizon in the care of the patients whose urticaria is not controlled with antihistamines. Recent international guidelines recommend omalizumab as the first choice of treatment for antihistamine-refractory CSU. However, as it is not curative neither disease-modifying agent, there is a subpopulation of CSU patients responding partly or never to omalizumab. The other things to be solved in the treatment of CU is that clinical evidence is still limited on chronic inducible urticaria (CIndU) and special populations. Thus, a new anti-IgE treatment, ligelizumab is actively evaluated in the efficacy compared with both placebo and omalizumab. Further understandings on the pathogenesis of CU can lead to the development of new mechanism-based therapeutics for CU patients.

Keywords: omalizumab, ligelizumab, IgE, urticaria, angioedema

1. Introduction

Symptomatic management to relieve itchy wheals has been recognized as the standard of care for chronic urticaria. However, around a half of patients with CU are refractory to recommended doses neither an increased doses of antihistamine. In these patients whose urticaria are not controlled with non-sedative antihistamines, more significantly impaired quality of life has been observed. Management guidelines for CU in past included omalizumab, cyclosporine, dapsone, hydroxychloroquine, methotrexate, montelukast, colchine, and phototherapy as alternative treatment for antihistamine-refractory CU [1, 2]. However, most of recent guidelines recommend omalizumab for the first of choice among various immunomodulating agents based on lots of study results [3, 4].

Omalizumab is the only biologics, approved for management of chronic spontaneous urticaria (CSU) in patients at age 12 years or older by Food and Drug Administration (FDA). It a recombinant humanized IgG1, monoclonal anti-IgE antibody. Although the pathophysiology of CU is not completely established, it is clear that mast cell activation is the key feature of CU. Omalizumab binds to free IgE at the Fc region and prohibits IgE from interacting with high-affinity receptor for Fc region of IgE (FcεRI) on mast cells, basophils and eosinophils [5, 6]. It has been shown to downregulate the expression of FcεRI on both mast cells and basophils [7]. This chapter reviews the current evidence of the efficacy, safety, and treatment response to biologics targeting IgE, including omalizumab, ligelizumab and quilizumab in CU patients.

2. Pivotal phase III trials with omalizumab in patients with CSU

The first successful use of omalizumab for CU was reported by Boyce in 2006 [8]. The 3 essential phase III multicenter, randomized, double-blinded studies that led to the FDA indication for CSU were the ASTERIA I [9] and II [10], and GLACIAL [11] trials. These trials included a total of 733 patients on omalizumab 75, 150, or 300 mg at 4-week intervals and 242 patients were allocated in the placebo groups. Clinical efficacy of omalizumab in randomized controlled trials including these 3 pivotal trials are summarized in **Table 1**.

ASTERIA I was a 40-week trial included patients receiving either omalizumab 75 mg, omalizumab 150 mg, omalizumab 300 mg, or placebo given in 4-week intervals for a 24-week treatment period with 16 weeks of follow-up [9]. The patients who had failed H1 antihistamine treatment at licenced doses were enrolled. All 3 doses of omalizumab met their primary efficacy endpoint of a reduction in weekly itch severity score (ISS) at 12 weeks compared with baseline (−6.46 with omalizumab 75 mg, −6.66 with omalizumab 150 mg, and − 9.40 with omalizumab 300 mg). The omalizumab 300 mg group achieved the minimally important difference in weekly ISS at a significantly shorter duration compared with the other omalizumab doses. However, urticaria symptoms returned to placebo levels after omalizumab was discontinued in all treatment groups during the follow-up period.

ASTERIA II was a 28-week trial that included 12 weeks of therapy with either omalizumab 75 mg, 150 mg, or 300 mg, or placebo in 4-week intervals with a 16-week follow-up period [10]. The patients having already failed treatment with approved doses of H1 antihistamines were included. The group of omalizumab 75 mg was failed to show significant difference in weekly ISS at 12 weeks compared with the placebo group. The omalizumab 150 mg and 300 mg groups reached significance for their primary end point of a mean change from baseline in weekly ISS at 12 weeks (−8.1 with omalizumab 150 mg and − 9.8 with omalizumab 300 mg), as compared with placebo. The proportion of patients who had complete symptom control was 16%, 22%, 44%, and 5% for omalizumab 75 mg, 150 mg, 300 mg, and placebo groups, respectively. During the 16-week follow-up period, the ISS for all omalizumab doses increased to levels similar to those of the placebo group.

GLACIAL trial included patients who had failed H1 antihistamines at up to 4 times the approved doses in addition to approved doses of leukotriene receptor antagonists or H2 antihistamines [11]. These patients were given either omalizumab 300 mg or placebo every 4 weeks for 24 weeks followed by a 16-week observation period. The weekly ISS at week 12 compared with baseline was significantly improved in the omalizumab 300 mg group compared with placebo (−8.6 with omalizumab 300 mg). All the other secondary efficacy end points also met

Trial name, Author, Year, Reference No.	Population	Study design	Intervention	Mean change from baseline in UAS7 (mean, 95% CI or SD)	No. of complete responders (% of UAS7 = 0)
MYSTIQUE Saini 2011 [12]	Patients aged 12–75 years with CU refractory to antihistamines.	Multicenter RDBPCT (N = 90; OMA75 = 23, OMA300 = 25, OMA600 = 21, placebo = 21)	Omalizumab 75, 300, 600 mg Single dose	Placebo: −6.9 (−11.5, 0.96) 75 mg: −9.8 (−17.77, −4.85) 300 mg: −19.9 (−25.4, −12.0) 600 mg: −14.6 (−22.5, −7.0) at 4 W	Placebo: 0% 75 mg: 4.4% 300 mg: 36.0% 600 mg: 28.6% at 4 W
XCUISITE Maurer 2011 [13]	Patients aged 18–70 years with a clinical diagnosis of moderate-to-severe CU.	Multicenter RDBPCT (N = 49; OMA = 27, placebo = 22)	Omalizumab 75 ~ 375 mg Q2W or Q4W based on the asthma dosing	Placebo: −7.9 300 mg: −17.8 at 24 W	Placebo: 4.5% 300 mg: 59.3% at 24 W
ASTERIA I Maurer 2013 [9]	Patients aged 12–75 years with moderate-to-severe CU who remained symptomatic despite H1AH.	Multicenter RDBPCT (N = 322; OMA75 = 82, OMA150 = 82, OMA300 = 79, placebo = 79)	Omalizumab 75, 150, 300 mg Q4W for 12 weeks	Placebo: −5.1 ± 5.6 75 mg: −5.9 ± 6.5 150 mg: −8.1 ± 6.4 300 mg: −9.8 ± 6.0 at 12 W	Placebo: 5% 75 mg: 16% 150 mg: 22% 300 mg: 53% at 12 W
ASTERIA II Saini 2015 [10]	Patients aged 12–75 years with a CU that remained symptomatic despite H1AH.	Multicenter RDBPCT (N = 318; OMA75 = 77, OMA150 = 80, OMA300 = 81, placebo = 80)	Omalizumab 75, 150, 300 mg Q4W for 24 weeks	Placebo: −8.01 ± 5.22 75 mg: −6.46 ± 6.14 150 mg: −6.66 ± 6.28 300 mg: −9.40 ± 5.73 at 12 W	Placebo: 8.8% 75 mg: 11.7% 150 mg: 15.0% 300 mg: 35.8% at 12 W
GLACIAL Kaplan 2013 [11]	Patients aged 12–75 years with a CU that remained symptomatic despite H1AH plus H2AH and/or LTRA.	Multicenter RDBPCT (post hoc analysis) (N = 336; OMA300 = 252, placebo = 84)	Omalizumab 300 mg Q4W for 24 weeks	Placebo: −8.5 (−11.1, −5.9) 300 mg: −19.0 (−20.6, −17.4) at 12 W Mean difference to placebo: −4.5 (−6.1, −3.0) at 24 W	34% vs. 5% at 12 W
X-ACT Staubach 2016 [14]	Patients aged 18–75 years with CSU and ≥ 4 episodes of angioedema who were symptomatic despite H1AH.	Multicenter RDBPCT (N = 91; OMA300 = 44, placebo = 47)	Omalizumab 300 mg Q4W for 24 weeks	Placebo: −6.5 ± 13.4 300 mg: −16.8 ± 14.8 Mean difference to placebo: −10.3 (−16.2, −3.9) at 28 W	50% vs. 10.6% at 28 W

Trial name, Author, Year, Reference No.	Population	Study design	Intervention	Mean change from baseline in UAS7 (mean, 95% CI or SD)	No. of complete responders (% of UAS7 = 0)
MoA Metz 2017 [15]	Patients aged 18–75 years with CU refractory to antihistamines.	Multicenter RDBPCT (N = 30; OMA300 = 20, placebo = 10)	Omalizumab 300 mg Q4W for 12 weeks	Placebo: −3.8 ± 6.63 300 mg: −11.4 ± 6.53 Mean difference to placebo: −14.82 at 12 W	NA
Jörg 2018 [17]	Patients aged 18–70 years with CSU refractory to H1AH.	Monocenteric RDBPCT Post hoc analysis (N = 30; OMA300 = 20, placebo = 10)	Omalizumab 300 mg Q4W for 16 weeks	NA	47.1% vs. 0% at 12 W 23.5% vs. 12.5% at 20 W
POLARIS Hide 2017 [19]	Japanese and Korean patients aged 12–75 years with CSU refractory to conventional H1AH at the randomization.	Multicenter RDBPCT (N = 218; OMA150 = 71, OMA300 = 73, placebo = 74)	Omalizumab 150, 300 mg Q4W for 12 weeks	Placebo: −13.9 150 mg: −18.8 300 mg: −22.4 at 12 W	Placebo: 4.1% 150 mg: 18.6% 300 mg: 35.6% at 12 W
XTEND-CIU Maurer 2018 [16] Casale 2019 [18]	Patients aged 12–75 years who remain symptomatic despite optimized H1AH treatment.	Multicenter RDBPCT (N = 134; OMA300 = 81, placebo = 53)	Omalizumab 300 mg Q4W for the 1st 24 W, and then randomized to OMA300 or placebo for additional 24 W	NA	36.8% at 12 W 52.0% at 24 W

Table 1.
Clinical efficacy of omalizumab in randomized controlled trials.

significance for the omalizumab group including change in weekly urticaria activity score (UAS7), Dermatology Life Qualirty Index, and proportion of patients who were itch and hive free. As with both ASTERIA trials, the effects of omalizumab appeared not to be permanent, and weekly ISS increased to placebo levels after discontinuing omalizumab treatment.

Recently, several systematic analyses based on various randomized controlled trials [9–19] to evaluate the effects of omalizumab for patients with CSU have been reported [3, 20–22]. These systematic reviews have provided high-quality of evidence on that omalizumab is effective in the treatment of antihistamine-refractory CSU independent of monthly dose [3, 22]. The dosage of 300 mg every 4 weeks is found to achieve better results in reductions of disease activity scores and in improvement of disease-specific quality of life. However, a recent meta-analysis analyzed minimal important differences in urticaria outcome measures, such as UAS7, ISS7, and quality of life demonstrated that omalizumab 300 mg resulted in clinically meaningful improvement of all the outcome measures, whereas omalizumab 150 mg failed to prove clinically meaningful improvement in any of them as compared with standard of care [20].

3. Optimal dosing and interval of omalizumab treatment

In patients with allergic asthma, optimal dose of omalizumab is determined by serum total IgE levels and body weight of the patients. Unlike for allergic asthma, the FDA approved omalizumab for the management of CSU at doses independent of serum IgE levels or body weight. Based on the 3 pivotal trials, [9–11] the approved doses of omalizumab is 150 mg or 300 mg every 4 weeks. Doses lower than 150 mg did not consistently show a significant improvement in efficacy compared with placebo, and the higher dose of 300 mg dependably showed faster and more robust efficacy. Interestingly, higher doses of omalizumab at 600 mg were explored in the dose-ranging single omalizumab dose phase II MYSTIQUE trial [23, 24]. Although no significant difference in changes of UAS7 at week 4 from baseline between the omalizumab 600 mg and 300 mg groups, there was also no increase in adverse events [25–27]. Cases of patients requiring higher than approved doses, up to 600 mg, to reach complete remission have been reported [25, 27].

4. Proper duration of omalizumab treatment

As shown in all phase III trials, cessation of omalizumab resulted in an increase in weekly itch and wheal scores and returning to placebo levels within 16 weeks [9–11]. These results indicate that omalizumab is effective in controlling symptoms, but they do not provide evidence that omalizumab induces remission from CSU. Therefore, longer durations of treatment may be required for some patients. Omalizumab shows very good safety efficacious at therapeutic durations of more than 1 year [23, 24]. As soon as patients achieved complete control, antihistamines can be tapered off [4].

Several strategies have been proposed for weaning including reduction monthly doses or lengthening the time between doses [28]. A patient-tailored tapering protocol on the basis of a patient's UAS7 scores while on omalizumab treatment is needed. Increase the injection interval by 1-week intervals can be recommended when the patient achieved a complete response to omalizumab after 6 months of treatment [29]. If a patient can tolerate every 8-week injections over a 4-month period without increased activity, these patients can often have omalizumab discontinued. Fortunately, most of patients who have experienced relapsed urticaria after stopping omalizumab treatment, respond well to retreatment of omalizumab with previously effective dose and interval [30, 31].

5. Predictors of the response to omalizumab treatment

In patients with CU, omalizumab is not a disease-modifying or curative treatment. The treatment response to omalizumab in patients with CU is classified according to the onset and extent of the response. Fast or early response is defined when the onset of therapeutic response to omalizumab in CU patients starts within the first 4 weeks. On the other hand, the response appearing gradually by weeks 12–16 weeks is defined as slow or late response. The extent of therapeutic response to omalizumab is based on the UAS7. Complete response includes the patients who achieve UAS7 = 0, no itch and wheal or UAS7 ≤ 6, well-controlled urticaria or have a significant improvement in UAS7 reduction from baseline (> 90%). Partial response is defined as UAS7 reduction between 30% and 90%. No response means that UAS7 reduction is less than 30% from baseline or the exacerbation of itchy wheals during omalizumab treatment [32, 33].

Around 70% of patients with CSU who benefit from omalizumab respond within the first week of treatment. From the results of 3 pivotal phase III trials, at week 4, well-controlled urticaria (UAS7 ≤ 6) was reported by 2 ~ 5%, 12 ~ 15%, 21 ~ 28%, and 37 ~ 51% of patients receiving placebo, 75, 150, 300 mg of omalizumab, respectively. And early response is linked to type I autoimmunity or IgE autoantibodies, such as IgE to thyroid persoxidase [13]. The proportion of well-controlled urticaria and complete responders during the 12-week of active treatment increased continuously. With continuous dosing of omalizumab 300 mg from 12 weeks to 24 weeks in ASTERIA I [9] and GLACIAL, [11] around a half of patients who did not respond at week 12 achieved complete response at week 24. The median time to complete response was also dependent on the dose of omalizumab. It was noted between 8 and 10 weeks for 300 mg of omalizumab, whereas fewer than 50% of patients in the 75 mg or 150 mg of omalizumab groups achieved complete response within the 12-week of treatment. However, around 40 ~ 50% of patients had partly or uncontrolled urticaria even with an active treatment of omalizumab for 24 weeks. Thus, before determining non-responders to omalizumab treatment and considering other therapeutics, use of omalizumab for at least 6 months is needed.

There are no markers to predict when their CSU will go into remission. Despite older and higher disease activity at onset, being female, and hypersensitivity to nonsteroidal anti-inflammatory drugs, comorbid CIndU, presence of angioedema, and thyroid disease were all reported to be associated with longer urticaria duration in CSU patients, [29] however, none on these markers guides to decide when to discontinue omalizumab.

Lower levels of serum total IgE at baseline (< 40 IU/mL) and decreased ratio of IgE levels at 4 weeks by baseline levels (<2.0) have been associated with higher risk of non-responder to omalizumab treatment in CSU patients [34]. Positive response to diagnostic tests for type IIb autoimmunity including basophil histamine releasability assay, autologous serum skin test, and anti-FcεRI autoantibody in the sera from CSU patients are regarded as indicators for slow or poor response to omalizumab [34, 35].

Studies evaluating the efficacy of up-dosing of omalizumab to 450 mg or 600 mg in a month revealed a comparable benefit for CSU patients with partial or non-response to 300 mg of omalizumab [26, 27, 36]. There also reports that shortening the injection interval can lead to complete response inpatients with partial or no response to omalizumab 300 mg every 4 weeks. The most recent guidelines recommend cyclosporine add-on as a fourth-line treatment in CSU patients whose urticaria is not controlled with omalizumab treatment [3, 4, 37].

6. Omalizumab treatment for chronic inducible urticaria

As chronic inducible urticaria (CIndU), induced by common physical stimuli including exposure to cold or heat, skin friction or pressure, sunlight, and exercise, with longer duration, difficult to avoid the offending trigger, CIndU affects severely patients' quality of life. A recent study reported that up to 76% of CSU patients were found to have a concurrent CIndU and these patients have more severe urticaria [38]. While omalizumab has been used to successfully treat CSU on the basis of strong evidence from randomized controlled trials, real-life studies, and meta-analyses, omalizumab is not yet licensed for CIndU.

A meta-analysis reported recently that omalizumab has substantial benefits in patients with various CIndUs [16]. Variation of omalizumab use was seen between the CIndU subtypes, with the strongest evidence available in patients with symptomatic dermographism (complete or partial response in 38/54 patients), cold urticaria (complete/partial response in 41/51 patients), and solar urticaria (complete/partial response in 28/36 patients). Little or no evidence was available on vibratory, aquagenic and contact urticaria.

A randomized, placebo-controlled trial involving 55 patients with symptomatic dermographism revealed that significant improvement in critical friction thresholds after 10 weeks of treatment with omalizumab 150 mg and 300 mg, compared with the placebo group [39]. No significant difference in efficacy was observed between omalizumab 150 mg and 300 mg groups. After 10 weeks of treatment, 6 (33%) of 18 receiving 150 mg of omalizumab and 8 (42%) of 19 patients receiving 300 mg of omalizumab did not respond at all compared with 15 (83%) of 18 in the placebo group. A retrospective observational study showed 86% of patients achieved a complete response [32].

Cold urticaria is the second most prevalent physical urticaria. A randomized, placebo-controlled trial including 31 patients with cold urticaria demonstrated significant clinical superiority of omalizumab versus placebo [40]. Mean changes in critical temperature threshold after 10 weeks of treatment were significantly higher in the omalizumab 150 mg and 300 mg groups compared with the placebo group. Improvements were seen by week 4. No significant dose-dependent response between the omalizumab 150 mg and 300 mg groups. After 10 weeks of treatment, 10% of 10 patients receiving omalizumab 150 mg and 22% of 9 patietns receiving 300 mg of omalizumab were non-responders compared with 75% of 12 patients in the placebo group.

Due to a longer symptomatic episode and a subtype of frequently accompanied in patients with CSU, delayed pressure urticaria was reported to result in a significant impairment of quality of life than other types of CIndU [41]. Furthermore, it is difficult to control delayed pressure urticatia with up-dosing of antihistamine treatment [16]. In a meta-analysis that found 11 publications of omalizumab treatment for patients with delayed pressure urticaria, favorable results were obtained [16]. Starting with 150 mg of omalizumab, 60% ~ 88% of patients with delayed pressure urticatia achieved complete control within 2 days.

There is sparse data on the efficacy of omalizumab for patients with cholinergic urticaria. Among retrospective analyses, one from the Germany [32] reported 62% of complete response and 25% of no response assessed by provocation test, whereas another study reported from Korean populations [42] showed relatively lower complete responders (4.8%, 1 of 21 patients).

Taken together, although evidence of the efficacy of omalizumab in CIndU has been accumulating, more data from randomized controlled trials are needed to establish the dose, injection interval, and treatment duration according to the type of CIndU. To date, while many studies proved a lower dose of 150 mg was enough to reach a good response, however as like in CSU patients, increasing dose of omalizumab in some patients with CIndU had better response. Most of studies found that CIndU patients achieved complete symptom control after the first injection of omalizumab, however, once discontinued, all patients got worse within 8 weeks after the last injection to need retreatment of omalizumab because antihistamines did not work for these patients [16].

7. Omalizumab treatment for angioedema

In X-ACT (Xolair Effects on Angioedema in Chronic Spontaneous Urticaria Treatment) study, a phase III, randomized, double-blind study involving selectively CSU patients with angioedema and wheals, omalizumab was superior to placebo in improving CU-Q2oL scores and reduction in angioedema-burdened days by three times during the 28-week of treatment [14, 43]. Angioedema was a prevalent symptom in patients with CSU in the three pivotal phase 3 studies of omalizumab and occurred in 44–53% of patients at baseline [9–11]. Treatment with 300 mg of omalizumab was efficacious in reducing patient-reported angioedema in patients with CIU/CSU who were symptomatic despite a variety of treatments [44]. Urgert et al. evaluated systematically the efficacy of omalizumab in CSU patients accompanying angioedema using 5 studies [21]. They provided high quality evidence of that the proportion of angioedema-free days were higher in the omalizumab group compared with placebo as well as use of rescue medications from baseline was significantly reduced in the omalizumab 300 mg group.

8. Omalizumab treatment for special populations

Although ASTERIA II [10] and GLACIAL [11] did include patients with 12 years and older, none of these larger trials addressed the use of omalizumab in the pediatric population below this age. Although significantly less common in the pediatric population, CU affects 0.1% to 0.3% of children with a similar morbidity profile as the adult population. A case series of the use of omalizumab for CU in the 4 patients in age from 4 to 16 years found that all 4 patients obtained complete response to omalizumab 150 mg monthly for the younger ones (age 4 and 5 years) and 300 mg monthly for the older patients at 10 and 16 years without any reported adverse events [45].

The EXPECT study evaluated the use of omalizumab during pregnancy [46]. In total, 191 pregnant women were included who had moderate to severe asthma and received at least 1 dose of omalizumab 8 weeks before conception or at any time during pregnancy. Based on the known outcomes of 169 pregnancies, there was no significant difference in spontaneous abortion, major congenital anomalies, prematurity, or low birth weight compared with a similar asthma population reported in previous studies [47, 48]. Because of the small number of patients in the study, it is difficult to draw any conclusions of safety on the use of omalizumab during pregnancy for CU [28]. Further studies are needed with larger sample sizes.

9. Safety issues of omalizumab

Safety was closely evaluated in all the randomized phase III trials [9–11]. ASTERIA II reported more headaches in the omalizumab 150 mg group compared with placebo but otherwise had no significant differences in adverse events. The GLACIAL study [11] showed no significant difference in adverse events between omalizumab group and placebo but did have some system-specific differences. In ASTERIA I, [9] headaches, arthralgia, and injection-site reactions were more common in the omalizumab groups but there was no significant difference in serious adverse events. No deaths, malignancies, or anaphylactic episodes were reported in these trials due to omalizumab.

Overall, omalizumab is very well tolerated and adverse reactions occurred in patients taking omalizumab were compatible with those on placebo in prospective, randomized trials for CU [3, 20, 49–51]. The most seriously considered adverse reaction is anaphylaxis-related to omalizumab that is defined as a combination of angioedema of the throat or tongue, bronchospasm, hypotension, syncope, and/or urticaria [52]. Omalizumab joint task force reviewed clinical trials and postmarketing surveillance data on omalizumab-induced anaphylaxis or anaphylactoid reactions [53]. They found a total of 35 patients with 42 episodes of anaphylaxis-related to omalizumab injection. Considering a total of 39510 patients who had exposed once to omalizumab, they estimated an anaphylaxis-reporting rate of 0.09% of patients [53]. The risk of anaphylaxis in patients with CU appears to be less than in those treated for asthma. In addition, there does not seem to be a dose-related effect on adverse events.

10. Anti-IgE therapeutics under development

10.1 Ligelizumab

Ligelizumab (QGE031) is a new promising humanizaed monoclonal anti-IgE antibody under development for the treatment of CSU patients. It has a 40-fold to 50-fold greater affinity to IgE compared with omalizumab [54]. In a phase 2b multicenter randomized placebo controlled trial, patients with antihistamine-refractory CSU were randomized to placebo, 300 mg of omalizumab, or 24, 72, or 240 mg of ligelizumab administered by subcutaneous injection with 4-week interval for 20 weeks [55]. Ligelizumab demonstrated rapid onset of action, dose-dependent efficacy, and superiority to omalizumab. At 12 week, a total of 30%, 51%, and 42% of the patients treated with 24 mg, 72 mg, and 240 mg of ligelizumab, respectivity, had complete control of urticaria, as compared with 26% of the patients receiving omalizumab 300 mg and none in the placebo group. More than 50% of patients taking 240 mg of ligelizumab were complete responders, a response rate twice than that seen in the omalizumab group. Furthermore, the mean time to relapse after the last injection was 4 weeks for omalizumab vs. 10 weeks for ligelizumab. Except higher rates of mild injection site reactions in the 240 mg of ligelizumab group, no difference in safety profiles of placebo, omalizumab, and ligelizumab was observed. The most frequently reported adverse events were viral upper respiratory tract infection and headache. No deaths or anaphylaxis events were reported in any of the trial groups. On the basis of favorable response of ligelizumab with a rapid onset of action, improved and sustained efficacy in antihistamine-refractory CSU patients over 300 mg of omalizumab treatment, now two phase III, multi-center, randomized, double-blind, active- and placebo-controlled, parallel-group studies (PEARL 1 and 2) are running. The primary outcome of these two trials will measure absolute change from baseline in UAS7 at Week 12 [56].

10.2 Quilizumab

Quilizumab, a humanized, afucosylated, monoclonal IgG1 antibody, binds membrane IgE at the M1-prime segment, which is absent in soluble IgE. In animal studies, quilizumab bound membrane IgE on IgE-switched B cells and plasmablasts and depleted them through apoptosis and antibody-dependent cell-mediated cytotoxicity [57]. In clinical trials, quilizumab reduced serum total and specific IgE levels in healthy volunteers and in patients with allergic rhinitis or mild asthma [58].

However, because quilizumab did not provide a significant differences in the clinical endpoints compared with placebo, it was indicated that ongoing IgE switching and stimulation of B-cell memory may not be key disease drivers [59].

11. Conclusion

Therapeutics modulating IgE levels and activities provide an efficient and very tolerable add-on treatment for patients with antihistamine-refractory CU. With a strong evidence of the efficacy and safety, omalizumab is recommended as the first choice of treatment for CSU patients who still suffered from urticaria with up-dosing antihistamine treatment in recent international guidelines. However, as it is not disease-modifying agent, there is a subpopulation of CSU patients responding incompletely or never to omalizumab. Moreover, clinical evidence on chronic inducible urticaria (CIndU) and special populations, such as children and older patients is still not enough. Thus, a new anti-IgE treatment, ligelizumab is actively evaluated in the efficacy compared with both placebo and omalizumab. Further understandings on the pathogenesis of CU can lead to the development of new mechanism-based therapeutics for CU patients.

Acknowledgements

This work was supported by a grant from the National Research Foundation of Korea (NRF) funded by the Korea government (MSIP) (NRF-2018R1A2B6006199) and a grant from the Korea Health Technology R&D Project through the Korea Health Industry Development Institute (KHIDI), funded by the Ministry of Health & Welfare, Republic of Korea (HI16C0992).

Conflict of interest

The authors declare no conflict of interest.

Author details

Young-Min Ye
Ajou University School of Medicine, Suwon, Korea

*Address all correspondence to: ye9007@ajou.ac.kr

References

[1] Bernstein JA, Lang DM, Khan DA, Craig T, Dreyfus D, Hsieh F, et al.: The diagnosis and management of acute and chronic urticaria: 2014 update. J Allergy Clin Immunol 2014;133:1270-1277.

[2] Zuberbier T: A summary of the new international eaaci/ga (2) len/edf/wao guidelines in urticaria. World Allergy Organ J 2012;5:S1-S5.

[3] Choi JH, Lee DH, Song WJ, Choi M, Kwon JW, Kim GW, et al.: The kaaaci/kda evidence-based practice guidelines for chronic spontaneous urticaria in korean adults and children: Part 2. Management of h1-antihistamine-refractory chronic urticaria. Allergy Asthma Immunol Res 2020;12:750-770.

[4] Zuberbier T, Aberer W, Asero R, Abdul Latiff AH, Baker D, Ballmer-Weber B, et al.: The eaaci/ga(2)len/edf/wao guideline for the definition, classification, diagnosis and management of urticaria. Allergy 2018;73:1393-1414.

[5] Beck LA, Marcotte GV, MacGlashan D, Togias A, Saini S: Omalizumab-induced reductions in mast cell fce psilon ri expression and function. J Allergy Clin Immunol 2004;114:527-530.

[6] Chang TW, Shiung YY: Anti-ige as a mast cell-stabilizing therapeutic agent. J Allergy Clin Immunol 2006;117:1203-1212; quiz 1213.

[7] Prussin C, Griffith DT, Boesel KM, Lin H, Foster B, Casale TB: Omalizumab treatment downregulates dendritic cell fcepsilonri expression. J Allergy Clin Immunol 2003;112:1147-1154.

[8] Boyce JA: Successful treatment of cold-induced urticaria/anaphylaxis with anti-ige. J Allergy Clin Immunol 2006;117:1415-1418.

[9] Maurer M, Rosen K, Hsieh HJ, Saini S, Grattan C, Gimenez-Arnau A, et al.: Omalizumab for the treatment of chronic idiopathic or spontaneous urticaria. N Engl J Med 2013;368:924-935.

[10] Saini SS, Bindslev-Jensen C, Maurer M, Grob JJ, Bulbul Baskan E, Bradley MS, et al.: Efficacy and safety of omalizumab in patients with chronic idiopathic/spontaneous urticaria who remain symptomatic on h1 antihistamines: A randomized, placebo-controlled study. J Invest Dermatol 2015;135:925.

[11] Kaplan A, Ledford D, Ashby M, Canvin J, Zazzali JL, Conner E, et al.: Omalizumab in patients with symptomatic chronic idiopathic/spontaneous urticaria despite standard combination therapy. J Allergy Clin Immunol 2013;132:101-109.

[12] Saini S, Rosen KE, Hsieh HJ, Wong DA, Conner E, Kaplan A, et al.: A randomized, placebo-controlled, dose-ranging study of single-dose omalizumab in patients with h1-antihistamine-refractory chronic idiopathic urticaria. J Allergy Clin Immunol 2011;128:567-573 e561.

[13] Maurer M, Altrichter S, Bieber T, Biedermann T, Bräutigam M, Seyfried S, et al.: Efficacy and safety of omalizumab in patients with chronic urticaria who exhibit ige against thyroperoxidase. Journal of Allergy and Clinical Immunology 2011;128:202-209. e205.

[14] Staubach P, Metz M, Chapman-Rothe N, Sieder C, Brautigam M, Canvin J, et al.: Effect of omalizumab on angioedema in h1 -antihistamine-resistant chronic spontaneous urticaria patients: Results from x-act, a randomized controlled trial. Allergy 2016;71:1135-1144.

[15] Metz M, Staubach P, Bauer A, Brehler R, Gericke J, Kangas M, et al.: Clinical efficacy of omalizumab in chronic spontaneous urticaria is associated with a reduction of fcepsilonri-positive cells in the skin. Theranostics 2017;7:1266-1276.

[16] Maurer M, Metz M, Brehler R, Hillen U, Jakob T, Mahler V, et al.: Omalizumab treatment in patients with chronic inducible urticaria: A systematic review of published evidence. J Allergy Clin Immunol 2018;141:638-649.

[17] Jorg L, Pecaric-Petkovic T, Reichenbach S, Coslovsky M, Stalder O, Pichler W, et al.: Double-blind placebo-controlled trial of the effect of omalizumab on basophils in chronic urticaria patients. Clin Exp Allergy 2018;48:196-204.

[18] Casale TB, Murphy TR, Holden M, Rajput Y, Yoo B, Bernstein JA: Impact of omalizumab on patient-reported outcomes in chronic idiopathic urticaria: Results from a randomized study (xtend-ciu). J Allergy Clin Immunol Pract 2019;7:2487-2490 e2481.

[19] Hide M, Park HS, Igarashi A, Ye YM, Kim TB, Yagami A, et al.: Efficacy and safety of omalizumab in japanese and korean patients with refractory chronic spontaneous urticaria. J Dermatol Sci 2017;87:70-78.

[20] Agache I, Rocha C, Pereira A, Song Y, Alonso-Coello P, Sola I, et al.: Efficacy and safety of treatment with omalizumab for chronic spontaneous urticaria: A systematic review for the eaaci biologicals guidelines. Allergy 2021;76:59-70.

[21] Urgert MC, van den Elzen MT, Knulst AC, Fedorowicz Z, van Zuuren EJ: Omalizumab in patients with chronic spontaneous urticaria: A systematic review and grade assessment. Br J Dermatol 2015;173:404-415.

[22] Rubini NPM, Ensina LFC, Silva EMK, Sano F, Sole D: Effectiveness and safety of omalizumab in the treatment of chronic spontaneous urticaria: Systematic review and meta-analysis. Allergol Immunopathol (Madr) 2019;47:515-522.

[23] Ensina LF, de Lacerda AE, Machado LM, Camelo-Nunes I, Sole D: Long-term omalizumab therapy for refractory chronic spontaneous urticaria: A real-life experience. Ann Allergy Asthma Immunol 2015;115:536.

[24] Har D, Patel S, Khan DA: Outcomes of using omalizumab for more than 1 year in refractory chronic urticaria. Ann Allergy Asthma Immunol 2015;115:126-129.

[25] Metz M, Vadasz Z, Kocatürk E, Giménez-Arnau AM: Omalizumab updosing in chronic spontaneous urticaria: An overview of real-world evidence. Clin Rev Allergy Immunol 2020;59:38-45.

[26] Niemeyer-van der Kolk T, van Maaren MS, van Doorn MBA: Personalized omalizumab treatment improves clinical benefit in patients with chronic spontaneous urticaria. J Allergy Clin Immunol 2018;142:1992-1994.

[27] Kocatürk E, Deza G, Kızıltaç K, Giménez-Arnau AM: Omalizumab updosing for better disease control in chronic spontaneous urticaria patients. Int Arch Allergy Immunol 2018;177:360-364.

[28] Joshi S, Khan DA: The expanding field of biologics in the management of chronic urticaria. J Allergy Clin Immunol Pract 2017;5:1489-1499.

[29] Turk M, Carneiro-Leao L, Kolkhir P, Bonnekoh H, Buttgereit T, Maurer M: How to treat patients with chronic spontaneous urticaria with omalizumab:

Questions and answers. J Allergy Clin Immunol Pract 2020;8:113-124.

[30] Metz M, Ohanyan T, Church MK, Maurer M: Retreatment with omalizumab results in rapid remission in chronic spontaneous and inducible urticaria. JAMA dermatology 2014;150:288-290.

[31] Türk M, Yılmaz İ, Bahçecioğlu SN: Treatment and retreatment with omalizumab in chronic spontaneous urticaria: Real life experience with twenty-five patients. Allergology International 2018;67:85-89.

[32] Metz M, Ohanyan T, Church MK, Maurer M: Omalizumab is an effective and rapidly acting therapy in difficult-to-treat chronic urticaria: A retrospective clinical analysis. J Dermatol Sci 2014;73:57-62.

[33] Kaplan A, Ferrer M, Bernstein JA, Antonova E, Trzaskoma B, Raimundo K, et al.: Timing and duration of omalizumab response in patients with chronic idiopathic/spontaneous urticaria. J Allergy Clin Immunol 2016;137:474-481.

[34] Marzano AV, Genovese G, Casazza G, Fierro MT, Dapavo P, Crimi N, et al.: Predictors of response to omalizumab and relapse in chronic spontaneous urticaria: A study of 470 patients. J Eur Acad Dermatol Venereol 2019;33:918-924.

[35] Asero R, Ferrucci S, Casazza G, Marzano AV, Cugno M: Total ige and atopic status in patients with severe chronic spontaneous urticaria unresponsive to omalizumab treatment. Allergy 2019;74:1561-1563.

[36] Curto-Barredo L, Spertino J, Figueras-Nart I, Exposito-Serrano V, Guilabert A, Mele-Ninot G, et al.: Omalizumab updosing allows disease activity control in patients with refractory chronic spontaneous urticaria. Br J Dermatol 2018;179:210-212.

[37] Sanchez J, Alvarez L, Cardona R: Cyclosporine and omalizumab together: A new option for chronic refractory urticaria. J Allergy Clin Immunol Pract 2020;8:2101-2103.

[38] Sanchez J, Amaya E, Acevedo A, Celis A, Caraballo D, Cardona R: Prevalence of inducible urticaria in patients with chronic spontaneous urticaria: Associated risk factors. J Allergy Clin Immunol Pract 2017;5: 464-470.

[39] Maurer M, Schutz A, Weller K, Schoepke N, Peveling-Oberhag A, Staubach P, et al.: Omalizumab is effective in symptomatic dermographism-results of a randomized placebo-controlled trial. J Allergy Clin Immunol 2017;140:870-873 e875.

[40] Metz M, Schutz A, Weller K, Gorczyza M, Zimmer S, Staubach P, et al.: Omalizumab is effective in cold urticaria-results of a randomized placebo-controlled trial. J Allergy Clin Immunol 2017;140:864-867 e865.

[41] Poon E, Seed PT, Greaves MW, Kobza-Black A: The extent and nature of disability in different urticarial conditions. Br J Dermatol 1999;140:667-671.

[42] Kim JH, Park HS, Ye YM, Shin YS, Kang HR, Chung SJ, et al.: Omalizumab treatment in patients with cholinergic urticaria: A real-world retrospective study in korea. Allergy Asthma Immunol Res 2020;12:894-896.

[43] Staubach P, Metz M, Chapman-Rothe N, Sieder C, Brautigam M, Maurer M, et al.: Omalizumab rapidly improves angioedema-related quality of life in adult patients with chronic spontaneous

urticaria: X-act study data. Allergy 2018;73:576-584.

[44] Zazzali JL, Kaplan A, Maurer M, Raimundo K, Trzaskoma B, Solari PG, et al.: Angioedema in the omalizumab chronic idiopathic/spontaneous urticaria pivotal studies. Ann Allergy Asthma Immunol 2016;117:370-377 e371.

[45] Netchiporouk E, Nguyen CH, Thuraisingham T, Jafarian F, Maurer M, Ben-Shoshan M: Management of pediatric chronic spontaneous and physical urticaria patients with omalizumab: Case series. Pediatr Allergy Immunol 2015;26:585-588.

[46] Namazy J, Cabana MD, Scheuerle AE, Thorp JM, Jr., Chen H, Carrigan G, et al.: The xolair pregnancy registry (expect): The safety of omalizumab use during pregnancy. J Allergy Clin Immunol 2015;135:407-412.

[47] Blais L, Kettani FZ, Elftouh N, Forget A: Effect of maternal asthma on the risk of specific congenital malformations: A population-based cohort study. Birth Defects Res A Clin Mol Teratol 2010;88:216-222.

[48] Demissie K, Breckenridge MB, Rhoads GG: Infant and maternal outcomes in the pregnancies of asthmatic women. Am J Respir Crit Care Med 1998;158:1091-1095.

[49] Zhao Z-T, Ji C-M, Yu W-J, Meng L, Hawro T, Wei J-F, et al.: Omalizumab for the treatment of chronic spontaneous urticaria: A meta-analysis of randomized clinical trials. Journal of Allergy and Clinical Immunology 2016;137:1742-1750. e1744.

[50] Giménez-Arnau AM: Omalizumab for treating chronic spontaneous urticaria: An expert review on efficacy and safety. Expert opinion on biological therapy 2017;17:375-385.

[51] Nettis E, Cegolon L, Di Leo E, Rizzini FL, Detoraki A, Canonica GW, et al.: Omalizumab chronic spontaneous urticaria: Efficacy, safety, predictors of treatment outcome, and time to response. Annals of Allergy, Asthma & Immunology 2018;121:474-478.

[52] Kim HL, Leigh R, Becker A: Omalizumab: Practical considerations regarding the risk of anaphylaxis. Allergy, asthma, and clinical immunology: official journal of the Canadian Society of Allergy and Clinical Immunology 2010;6:32-32.

[53] Cox L, Platts-Mills TA, Finegold I, Schwartz LB, Simons FER, Wallace DV: American academy of allergy, asthma & immunology/american college of allergy, asthma and immunology joint task force report on omalizumab-associated anaphylaxis. Journal of allergy and clinical immunology 2007;120:1373-1377.

[54] Gasser P, Tarchevskaya SS, Guntern P, Brigger D, Ruppli R, Zbären N, et al.: The mechanistic and functional profile of the therapeutic anti-ige antibody ligelizumab differs from omalizumab. Nature communications 2020;11:1-14.

[55] Maurer M, Gimenez-Arnau AM, Sussman G, Metz M, Baker DR, Bauer A, et al.: Ligelizumab for chronic spontaneous urticaria. N Engl J Med 2019;381:1321-1332.

[56] Wedi B: Ligelizumab for the treatment of chronic spontaneous urticaria. Expert opinion on biological therapy 2020;20:853-861.

[57] Hans DB, Yuwen LL, Zhonghua L, Martha T, Meng YG, Mercedesz B, et al.: Quilizumab is an afucosylated humanized anti-m1 prime therapeutic antibody. Clinical Anti-Inflammatory & Anti-Allergy Drugs (Discontinued) 2014;1:24-31.

[58] Scheerens H, Putnam W, Zheng Y, Wang Y, Mosesova S, Maciuca R, et al.: Treatment with memp1972a, an anti-m1 prime monoclonal antibody, reduced serum ige in healthy volunteers and patients with allergic rhinitis; in B33 asthma therapy: Novel approaches, American Thoracic Society, 2012, pp A6791-A6791.

[59] Harris JM, Cabanski CR, Scheerens H, Samineni D, Bradley MS, Cochran C, et al.: A randomized trial of quilizumab in adults with refractory chronic spontaneous urticaria. J Allergy Clin Immunol 2016;138:1730-1732.

Chapter 5

The Role of Anti-IgE Antibodies in Urticaria

Patrizia Pepe and Victor Desmond Mandel

Abstract

Chronic urticaria, a common mast cell driven disease, has been considered so far an underestimated and difficult to treat disease, very often resulting in high physical, psychological and socio-economic burden. More than 60% of these patients are unresponsive to second generation H1 antihistamines, the first-line symptomatic treatment for urticaria. However, anti-IgE drugs (omalizumab and ligelizumab) showed improved activity in urticaria-treated patients with inadequate symptom control. Omalizumab has been widely proven to be very effective and well-tolerated in patients with antihistamine-refractory chronic spontaneous urticaria and inducible urticaria and is currently licensed for these indication as third-line treatment. Ligelizumab, a next-generation monoclonal anti-IgE antibody with higher affinity to IgE compared to omalizumab and a similar safety profile, has recently demonstrated to be even more effective than omalizumab. This review is focused on the role of anti-IgE antibodies in chronic urticaria.

Keywords: Urticaria, Chronic Spontaneous Urticaria, Chronic Inducible Urticaria, Anti-IgE antibodies, Omalizumab, Ligelizumab

1. Introduction

Urticaria is a common mast cell-driven disease characterised by wheals (1–24 hours) and/or angioedema (up to 72 hours) (**Figure 1**), defined as acute when symptoms last <6 weeks or chronic if they occur continuously or intermittently for ≥6 weeks [1]. Approximately 50% of patients have both hives and angioedema, whereas 40% have wheals alone, and 10% have angioedema alone [2]. Moreover, Chronic Urticaria (CU) can be further classified as Chronic Inducible Urticaria (CIndU) when appear in response to specific eliciting factors, such as thermal agents, vibration, cholinergic factors, aquagenic, and delayed pressure or as Chronic Spontaneous Urticaria (CSU) if the above mentioned triggers have been excluded [1].

1.1 The prevalence of Chronic Urticaria

Both children and adults may develop urticaria, with the peak age of onset in adults being between 20 and 40 years [2]. The lifetime prevalence of Acute Urticaria (AU) ranges from <1% to 24% (12% to 24% in Europe), depending on the age range, method of sampling, and geographic location [3]. Instead, CU is estimated at 1% but there is no reliable data regarding its prevalence due to the lack of cross-sectional studies [4]. About 20% to 45% of patients with AU develop into CU.

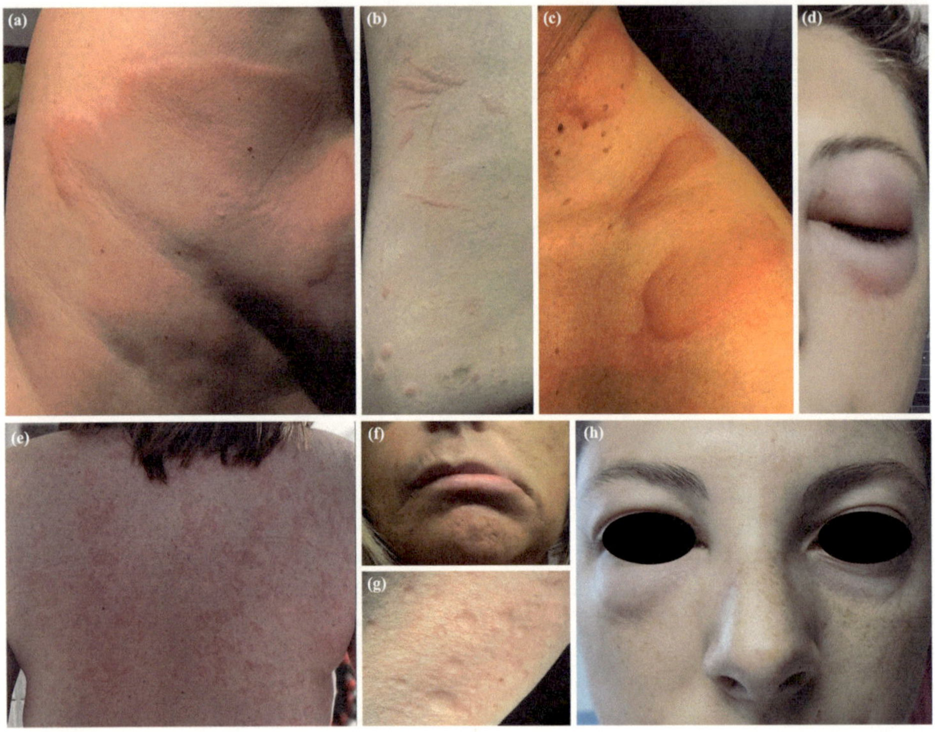

Figure 1.
(a–h): Urticaria is characterised by an outbreak of swollen, pale red bumps or plaques on the skin (wheals) and can also manifest as deep swelling around the eyes, lips, and face (angioedema) that appears suddenly.

CSU occurs in 0.5–1% of the population at any point in time, with its incidence peaking between 20 and 40 years of age [5]. CSU is considered more common in adults than in children and women are affected twice as often as men. However, recent studies have suggested that the prevalence of CSU in the paediatric population is similar to that of the adult population [6].

Finally, the CIndU prevalence is lower than other types of urticaria (e.g., acquired cold urticaria in Europe is extimated around 0.5%) [3].

1.2 The burden of Chronic Urticaria

In 1997 O'Donnel et al. compared the Quality of Life (QoL) scores in 142 patients with CU and 98 patients with life-threatening heart disease, finding similar QoL scores in both groups [7]. Indeed, many CU patients exhibit a severe impairment of their quality of life. The long disease duration (on average aorund two to five years) and the lack of curative therapy have been underlined as the two main aspects that contribute to the high physical, psychological and socio-economic burden of CU [8, 9]. The last EAACI/GA^2LEN/EDF/WAO guideline recommends "aiming at complete symptom control in urticaria, considering as much as possible the safety and the QoL of each individual patient" [1]. Currently, two specific QoL questionnaires are available for evaluating the burden of CU on patients: Chronic Urticaria Quality of Life (CU-Q2oL) and Angioedema Quality of Life (AE-QoL). Moreover, in order to collect quality, real-life data on CU patient characteristics, the course of disease, underlying causes, comorbidities, treatment responses, quality of life impairment and health care costs the Chronic Urticaria Registry was recently set up [10].

1.3 Patient-reported outcome measures in Chronic Urticaria

Patient-reported outcome measures are instruments of objective and subjective evaluation for the management of CU and are essential tools for assessing treatment effects in clinical trials.

As described above, CU-Q2oL and AE-QoL are the two questionnaires available for evaluating the CU burden on QoL. Instead, the Urticaria Control Test (UCT) is a valid and reliable tool to assess disease control in patients with CU and a score of ≥12 indicates well-controlled urticaria [1]. However, the most frequently utilized tool in clinical trials is the 7 days Urticaria Activity Score (UAS7) [1, 11]. It is also suitable for evaluation of disease activity by urticaria patients and their treating physicians. The UAS7 is based on the patient self-assessment of the two main urticaria signs and symptoms recorded once a day for 7 consecutive days:

- wheals: 0 = none; 1 = mild (<20 wheals/24 hours); 2 = moderate (20–50 wheals/24 hours); 3 = intense (>50 wheals/24 hours or large confluent areas of wheals);

- pruritus: 0 = none; 1 = mild (present but not annoying or troublesome); 2 = moderate (troublesome but does not interfere with normal daily activity or sleep); 3 = severe (severe pruritus, which is sufficiently troublesome to interfere with normal daily activity or sleep).

The sum of score is 0–6 for each day, and 0–42 for the UAS7 (0 = urticaria-free; 1–6 = well-controlled urticaria; 7–15 = mild activity; 16–27 = moderate activity; 28–42 = severe activity), respectively. Overall disease activity is best measured by advising patients to document 24-hour self-evaluation scores for several days.

For the patients affected by recurrent angioedema, alone or in addition to wheals, the last EAACI/GA^{2}LEN/EDF/WAO guideline also suggests to use the Angioedema Activity Score (AAS) [1]. It consists of five items regarding the characteristics of angioedema to have occurred in previous 24 hours [11]. A score between 0 and 3 is assigned to every answer field. The question scores are added up to produce a daily score (0–15). Daily AAS can be summed to give 7-day (0–105), 4-week (0–420), and 12-week scores (0–1260) [12].

1.4 The Chronic Urticaria treatment guidelines

As first-line symptomatic treatment for urticaria, the EAACI/GA^{2}LEN/EDF/WAO guideline suggests regular administration of second-generation, nonsedating, nonimpairing H1-receptor antihistamines due to their efficacy and good safety profile [1]. This class of drugs has a greater receptor specificity, lower penetration of the blood–brain barrier, and less likely to cause drowsiness or psychomotor impairment in comparison to the first-generation antihistamines.

In non-responders adult or paediatric patients, the second-line treatment is the up-dosing of the antihistamine by as much as 4-fold. For patients (aged 12 years and older) who have not responded to four-times the standard dose of second-generation H1-receptor antihistamine, omalizumab, a humanised monoclonal anti-IgE antibody, as add-on therapy is considered the third-line treatment. If there is no response to the omalizumab within 6 months, or if the condition is intolerable, the fourth-line treatment is the prescription of cyclosporine A (CsA), which inhibits the production of IL-2, IL-3, IL-4, and TNF-α in lymphocytes and the IgE-mediated release of histamine from mast cells. High doses of CsA and long duration treatment are associated with adverse events such as abdominal pain, nausea, vomiting, paresthesia, headache, hirsutism, elevated serum creatinine, and hypertension;

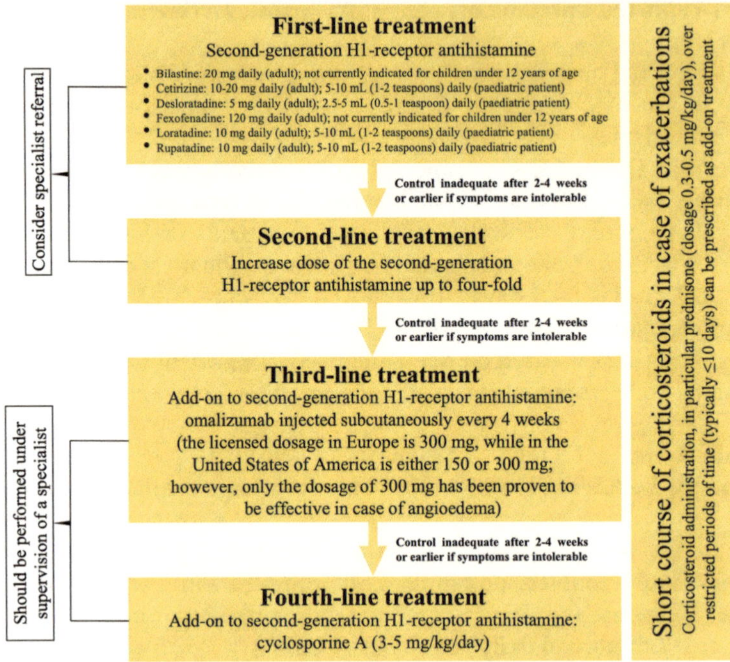

Figure 2.
Simplified stepwise algorithm for the treatment of urticaria adapted from the current EAACI/GA²LEN/EDF/WAO guideline.

however, these side effects resolve after reducing dosage [13]. Nevertheless, CsA should be avoided in patients with chronic kidney disease or poorly controlled hypertension. CsA at the dose of 3–5 mg/kg/day has been shown in small, double-blind, randomised controlled trials to be effective in patients with CSU who do not adequately respond to antihistamines [14, 15]. During CsA treatment, given the significant side effects, the blood pressure, renal function, and serum CsA levels should be monitored regularly.

A simplified stepwise algorithm for the treatment of CSU adapted from the EAACI/GA²LEN/EDF/WAO guideline is summarised in **Figure 2**. At any moment, short courses of corticosteroids (e.g. prednisone 25 mg/daily) are admitted if symptoms are exacerbated or poorly controlled [1].

1.5 The anthystamines limit in Chronic Spontaneous Urticaria

In the pre-omalizumab period, treating CSU patients was a real challenge for physicians due to the low rates of response to H1-antihistamines, which were the only approved medication and the mainstay of symptomatic treatment. Two meta-analysis including studies published between January 1990 and November 2014 revealed that 63.2% and 38.6% of patients remain symptomatic despite treatment with licensed dose and updosed H1-antihistamines, respectively [16]. Another study reported even lower response rates to standard dosage, with disease control in only 22% of patients [17].

2. The role of anti-IgE antibodies in Urticaria

The immune system is a network of cells, tissues, and organs that work together to defend the body against attacks by foreign invaders such as bacteria, viruses, parasites, and fungi [18]. The host uses both innate and adaptive mechanisms to detect and eliminate pathogenic microbes, and both of these mechanisms include self-nonself discrimination. Immunoglobulins (Ig), also known as antibodies, are glycoproteins produced by white blood cells that are specific for an antigen (e.g., bacteria, viruses, parasites, or fungi), aiding its destruction by a cascade of downstream pathways. There are five primary classes of Igs (IgG, IgM, IgA, IgD and IgE), which differ in their biological features, structure, target specificity, and distribution [19]. Among them, IgE are involved in allergic reactions with a type I autoimmune mechanism.

2.1 IgE

It is believed that IgE have evolved to protect humans from helminth infections, which are one of the major threats to human life. IgE molecules exist in a monomeric form consisting of two heavy and two light chains and are the most important participants in an allergic reaction [20]. When a foreign substance, called allergen, enters our body, a person with an inherited predisposition to this substance will begin to develop a specific type of IgE, which will evoke a cascade of reactions aimed to eliminating this allergen. IgE are present in serum at very low concentration (~50–200 ng/mL in a normal individual) and have a very short half-life (1–2 days). However, tissue-resident IgE may persist for several days (approximate half-life of 2 weeks in the skin) [21, 22]. This may be due to the extremely high affinity of IgE for the IgE Fc receptor (FcεRI) and in particular its slow dissociation from this receptor, resulting in re-binding of the dissociated IgE to its receptors, and restricted diffusion away from the tissue within which it resides [23].

There are two structurally and functionally distinct receptors that bind with the Fc epsilon (Fcε) region of IgE: the high affinity FcεRI and the lower affinity CD23 FcεRII [24, 25]. Through their Fc portions, IgE molecules bind to the Fc receptors present on the surface of mast cells and basophils. The cross-linking of such membrane-bound IgE antibodies by multivalent antigens triggers the release of chemically active substances, such as histamine, leukotrienes, prostaglandins, and chemotactic factors, from the cells. These substances initiate allergic and inflammatory reactions and serve as a chemoattractant for other cells [26].

2.2 Anti-IgE antibodies as Chronic Urticaria treatment: why?

This is the first question claimed by the scientific community, since IgE are involved in allergic reactions and CU is not known as an allergic reaction. Before answering this question, we should know the mechanism of action of omalizumab in CSU. Omalizumab has been effective in the treatment of urticaria, believed to have an autoimmune origin, and in cases where the etiology is unknown [27].

There are several hypotheses regarding the mechanism of action of omalizumab in CSU patients. One of them is based on the fact that the density of IgE receptors on the surface of mast cells and basophils is proportional to individual patient's plasma IgE levels [28, 29]. It is hypothesized that omalizumab, by lowering free IgE levels in the blood and subsequently in the skin, may lead to down-regulation of a large percentage of surface IgE receptors, thereby decreasing downstream signaling via the FcεRI receptor pathway [30, 31]. Cell activation would then be diminished, and subsequent inflammatory processes, as complement activation and cellular infiltration, would be suppressed as well. As a consequence, the frequency and severity of symptoms of CSU would be lessened [28, 30, 31].

Another hypothesis is that omalizumab reduces the levels of circulating IgE, leading to a rapid and non-specific desensitization of cutaneous mast cells [32].

Subsequent effects, such as down-regulation of IgE receptor, may help to sustain the response. Serrano-Candelas et al. demonstrated comparable actions of omalizumab on mast cells and basophils while investigating the in vitro mechanism of action of omalizumab on these cells [33].

In a review by Kaplan et al. new insights into the potential mechanisms of action contributing to the efficacy of omalizumab in CIndU/CSU have been suggested based on both clinical and in vitro studies [30]:

- omalizumab lowers IgE levels and down-regulates IgE receptors;
- reduces mast-cell releasability;
- decreases available FcεRI more slowly on mast cells than on basophils;
- reduces IgE+/FcεRI+ cells by ~12 weeks;
- reverses basopenia and improves basophil IgE receptor function;
- reduces the activity of intrinsically "abnormal" IgE;
- decreases the activity of IgG autoantibodies against FcεRI and IgE;
- reduces the activity of IgE autoantibodies against an antigen or autoantigen that has yet to be definitively identified;
- decreases in vitro coagulation abnormalities associated with disease activity.

Deza et al. investigated the effect of omalizumab on the basophil expression of FcεRI receptor in a cohort of patients with active CSU [34]. Patients exhibiting significant clinical improvement showed a sharp reduction in the levels of basophil FcεRI after 4 weeks ($p < 0.0001$), which was maintained throughout the total duration of the treatment.

In a study by Asero et al., omalizumab responders showed a dramatic decrease of D-dimer plasma levels after the first administration of the drug ($p = 0.003$), suggesting a possible effect of omalizumab on coagulation activation and fibrin degradation [32].

However, none of these theories fully account for the pattern of symptom improvement seen with omalizumab therapy. Therefore, additional research is warranted to further explain the involvement of omalizumab in relieving symptoms associated with the complex, multifactorial pathogenesis of CIndU/CSU.

2.3 The Chronic Spontaneous Urticaria main endotypes

CSU is a mast cell-driven disease. The initial event in the development of skin changes, such as sensory nerve stimulation, vasodilation and extravasation, as well as the recruitment of basophils, eosinophils, and T cells, which lead to whealing, itch, and angioedema is attributed to the degranulation of skin mast cells.

Two groups of mast cell degranulation signals have been so far identified and characterized in CSU pathogenesis: IgE autoantibodies to autoallergens and IgG autoantibodies that target activating mast cell receptors [30]. Therefore, it is now clear that there are at least 2 distinct pathways, type I and type IIb autoimmunity, that contribute to the pathogenesis of this complex disease [35]. In type I hypersensitivity to self, also called autoallergy, antigens crosslink the IgE on mast cells and basophils to cause release of vasoactive mediators, while in type IIb hypersensitivity antibodies, usually IgG, bind to antigen on a target cell.

About twenty years ago, the demonstration of IgE autoantibodies against the thyroid microsomal antigen thyroperoxidase in the serum of a CSU patient, identified a possible role of type I autoimmunity in the pathogenesis of urticaria [36]. Many studies have further characterized the prevalence and pathogenic relevance of type I autoimmunity in CSU. In particular, CSU patients were found to express more than 2-fold higher IgE-anti-thyroperoxidase serum levels as compared to healthy control subjects ($p < 0.001$) [37].

Kolkhir et al. systematically evaluated the literature on the prevalence of thyroid autoimmunity in CSU and vice-versa, finding a positive correlation between CSU and elevated levels of IgG antithyroid autoantibodies with the studies reporting rates consisted in 10% [38]. Levels of IgG against thyroid peroxidase resulted more often elevated in CSU than those of other IgG antithyroid autoantibodies (strong evidence). Moreover, CSU patients exhibited significantly higher levels of IgG antithyroid autoantibodies (strong evidence) and IgE anti-thyroperoxidase (weak evidence) than controls.

However, IgE autoantibodies directed to a large assortment of autoantigens beyond thyroperoxidase are expressed in the skin of CSU patients as thyroglobulin, tissue factor, and interleukin (IL)-24 [39, 40]. Hatada et al. found that the anti-dsDNA IgE levels were significantly higher in patients with CU than in normal subjects, while no differences in the anti-dsDNA IgG levels were observed [41]. Furthermore, most of the studies confirm that IgE autoantibodies should be responsible for the increased total IgE levels in CSU patients in which, differently to the control subjects, most of the IgE was found to be directed against autoantibodies.

A type IIb hypersensitivity mechanism in which IgG autoantibodies against IgE were involved, was first described in CSU in 1988 [42]. Few years later, IgG autoantibodies directed to FcεRI, the high-affinity receptor for IgE on masthocytes and basophils, were also identified [42]. Grattan et al. introduced the Autologous Serum Skin Test (ASST) in CSU patients, consisting in eliciting with an intradermal injection of their own serum a wheal and flare response [43]. A positive reaction in the ASST confirm the presence of these autoantibodies.

CSU driving by type IIb autoimmune mechanisms is further supported by the basophil activation test [44]. The serum of a subpopulation of CSU patients stimulates heterologous basophils and this activity is due to the presence of autoantibodies against FcεRI as well as in positive ASST responses.

The two endotypes play a key role in inducing different phenotipe of the same disease: type I (autoreactive) and type IIb (autoimmune) CSU patients differ in some features, laboratory markers, and rates and speed of response to treatment [45]. In particular, type IIb autoimmune CSU patients have been suggested to have higher disease activity and longer disease duration as well as higher rates of autoimmune comorbidity. Basopenia and eosinopenia may also be more common.

A higher proportion of patients receiving omalizumab 300 mg achieved response as early as week 4 (early responders) when compared with placebo [46]. This is in line with type I autoimmune/autoreactive mechanism: anti-IgE rapidly binds free IgE, including IgE against autoantigens, and IgE/anti-IgE complexes bind autoallergens preventing mast cell degranulation. CSU patients that take more than a month (late responders) to respond to omalizumab, probably underwent a type IIb autoimmunity, where the reduction of free IgE results in the slow loss of membrane-bound FcεRI from skin mast cells [46].

New endotypes of CSU have been proposed in addiction by recent reports, suggesting a key role of the coagulation pathway factors, ligands of the Mas-related

G protein–coupled receptor X2, basophils, and other signals in the pathogenesis of CSU [47, 48]. Moreover, other research to characterize better the role and the relevance of type I and type IIb autoimmunity in CSU and to support the existence of distinct and separate endotypes, are still in progress.

In contrast to CSU, autoimmunity in CIndU has not yet been described.

3. Omalizumab in Urticaria

Omalizumab is a recombinant deoxyribonucleic acid-derived humanized monoclonal antibody manufactured from a mammalian cell line, that selectively binds to IgE. The antibody is an IgG1 kappa that contains human framework regions with the complementary-determining regions of a murine parent antibody that binds to free IgE, preventing its interaction with FcεRI (**Table 1**). It has been firstly indicated for adults and children (6 years of age and above) with moderate to severe persistent allergic asthma. Ten years later, omalizumab has been approved for the treatment of adults and adolescents (12 years of age and above) with CSU refractory to standard of care.

3.1 Phase II and III clinical studies

Omalizumab preliminary dose selection was provided by the phase II study MYSTIQUE, which evaluated the effect of the drug at different dosages [49]. While these results provided the preliminary data, pivotal dose selection was ultimately evaluated in two pivotal phase III efficacy trials (ASTERIA I and ASTERIA II) and was supplemented by data from the safety trial (GLACIAL) [12]. The GLACIAL study was adequately designed and controlled to provide efficacy information as well.

The MYSTIQUE study assessed the efficacy of three doses of omalizumab (75 mg, 300 mg, and 600 mg) as a single subcutaneous injection in patients with CSU refractory to H1-antihistamines (n = 90), which was followed by a 12-week observation period [49]. The primary endpoint was the mean change in UAS7 at Week 4. Patients in the omalizumab 300 mg and 600 mg groups had significantly greater improvements from baseline in the scores of UAS7 and weekly Itch Severity Score (ISS) compared with those in the placebo group. No additional benefits were observed in the 600 mg group over the 300 mg group. UAS7 scores with omalizumab 75 mg showed only marginal differences versus placebo [50]. The most frequently reported (≥5%) treatment-emergent adverse effects (AEs) during the treatment period were upper respiratory tract infection, headache, nasopharyngitis, and dysmenorrhea. Most AEs were mild to moderate in severity and were considered not related to the study drug [49].

In the XCUISITE study, omalizumab was administered according to the dosing table for allergic asthma using baseline IgE level and weight [50]. Treatment effects were analyzed by individual dose levels for the primary endpoint (change from baseline in UAS7 after 24 weeks) [51]. In the groups receiving omalizumab 300 mg and 150 mg every 4 weeks, a considerable improvement was observed in the UAS7 score compared with that in the placebo group, with a more pronounced effect observed with 300 mg [12]. Although the results of the study suggested a dose–response relationship, no conclusions were made regarding the comparative efficacy between the dose levels since the number of patients in each group was small (n = 6–7) and participants were not randomly assigned to the different dose levels [52]. In terms of safety in the XCUISITE study, the overall incidence of AEs during the treatment period was similar between the omalizumab and placebo groups. The

DOI: http://dx.doi.org/10.5772/intechopen.97025

Anti-IgE Antibodies	Monoclonal antibody type	Equilibrium dissociation constant (K_D)	Pharmacokinetics	Mechanism of action	Administration	Adverse events (most frequent)
Omalizumab, Xolair® (E25, IGE025)	Humanized IgG1/κ-light chain	7×10^{-9} M	• Maximum serum concentration within 7–8 days • Terminal elimination half-life ≈24 days • Steady state serum concentration at week 12	• Attaches to the Cε3 domain of serum IgE, and thereby inhibits these IgE antibodies from binding to FcεRI high-affinity IgE receptor and CD23 receptor • No binding to receptor-bound IgE • Dissociates IgE from FcεRI	• 300 mg (two pre-filled syringes with 150 mg) subcutaneously • Every 4 weeks • Self-administration possible after four tolerated doses	• Injection-site reactions • Upper respiratory infection • Headache
Ligelizumab (QGE031)	Humanized, IgG1/κ-light chain	1.4×10^{-10} M	• Maximum serum concentration within 4 days • Terminal elimination half-life ≈20–25 days • Steady state serum concentration at week 8–16	• Inhibits IgE antibodies from binding to the FcεRI high-affinity IgE receptor • Interference with CD23 binding is debated • No binding to receptor-bound IgE, therefore no triggering of effector cells such as mast cells or basophils	• 120 mg / 240 mg subcutaneously • Every 4 weeks • Final dosing regimen has yet to be defined	• Injection-site reactions • Upper respiratory infection • Headache
UB-221	Humanized IgG1	Not published	Not published	• Attaches to the Cε3 domain of serum IgE, and thereby inhibits these IgE antibodies from binding to FcεRI high-affinity IgE receptor • No inhibition of the interaction between IgE and CD23 • No binding to FcεRI-bound IgE, but binding to CD23-bound IgE, down-regulates IgE synthesis	• 0.2 / 0.6 / 2 / 6 / 10 mg/kg intravenously • Single dose • Final dosing regimen has yet to be defined	Not published
Quilizumab	Humanized, afucosylated, IgG1/κ-light chain	Not published	• Mean maximum observed serum concentrations of 34 ± 12.6 μg/mL at time of maximum observed serum concentration of 36.2 ± 3.5 days • Terminal elimination half-life ≈19–21 days	• Binds membrane IgE at the M1-prime segment • No binding to free IgE	• 300 mg subcutaneously • Every 4 weeks	• Injection-site reactions • Arthralgia • Headache

Table 1.
Summary of the Anti-IgE Antibodies in Chronic Urticaria.

most frequent AEs (>5%) in both groups were diarrhea, nasopharyngitis, and headache. No severe AEs or deaths related to omalizumab were reported [51].

The ASTERIA I, ASTERIA II, and GLACIAL studies were part of the omalizumab registration program in CSU. These were phase III, randomized, multicenter, double-blind, placebo-controlled studies that evaluated the efficacy and safety of omalizumab in patients with CSU [52–54]. Patients with CSU who remained symptomatic despite H1-antihistamine therapy were randomized to receive either placebo or subcutis omalizumab at the dosage of 75 mg, 150 mg, or 300 mg every 4 weeks for a total of 24 weeks in ASTERIA I (n = 319) and 12 weeks in ASTERIA II (n = 323) [52, 53]. The primary endpoint in both trials was the mean change in the ISS score at Week 12. Secondary was to evaluate the variation from baseline to Week 12 in the UAS7 score, weekly number of hives score, median time to minimally important difference in the ISS, weekly size of the largest hive score, proportion of patients with UAS7 $\leq$ 6, change in the Dermatology Life Quality Index score, proportion of patients with UAS7 = 0, and proportion of angioedema-free days from Week 4 to Week 12.

Instead, GLACIAL (n = 336) primarily evaluated the safety of omalizumab in patients with CSU who remained symptomatic despite treatment with H1-antihistamines (at up to four times the approved dose) plus H2-antihistamines and/or leukotriene receptor antagonists [51], according to the EAACI/GA^{2}LEN/EDF/WAO urticaria guideline at that time [1]. In this study, patients were randomized 3:1 to receive either subcutaneous omalizumab 300 mg every 4 weeks or placebo for 24 weeks.

In all three studies, the treatment period was followed by a 16-week observation period during which no treatment was given [52]. Overall, no new safety issues were identified in the CSU clinical program [51]. No deaths occurred during either trial. The pivotal efficacy trials demonstrated a consistent dose-dependent treatment effect for the evaluated endpoints [49].

Anyway the licensed dosage for omalizumab for refractory CSU, with or without angioedema, in Europe is 300 mg every 4 weeks, independent of patient body weight, body mass index or serum IgE level, while in the USA this is either 150 or 300 mg [12, 52]. Instead, only the dosage of 300 mg every 4 weeks has been proven to be effective in case of angioedema. Currently, the licensed dosage in Italy is 300 mg every 4 weeks over a 6-month period, and in the case of disease recurrence, a minimum of 8 weeks suspension from omalizumab is mandatory, and then it can be prescribed again for a further 5 months only [12]. This schedule (6 months treatment, 8 weeks suspension, and 5 months therapy) can be repeated for eventual relapses; however, this de novo treatment is considered off-label.

To date, there are no licensed treatment options for CIndU and the recommended dosage with omalizumab is similar to CSU.

3.2 Omalizumab: real-life evidences

In clinical settings, the treatment of refractory CSU with omalizumab has been shown to be similar to, or in some cases even better than, those reported by the pivotal randomized controlled trials [12, 55–61].

The retrospective analysis of the three pivotal studies (ASTERIA I, ASTERIA II, and GLACIAL) put first in evidence that some CSU patients respond to treatment more quickly than others and for this reason two different categories were identified: "fast responders" for those who respond within 4–6 weeks and "slow responders" for whom obtain a response more gradually (from 12 to 16 weeks) [12]. However, "slow responders" may still respond even after 24 weeks, while some "fast responders" may obtain a response to treatment within 1 week, suggesting that the response patterns of patients to omalizumab may be due to the different pathomechanisms of the disease. These two different patterns of response have been soon confirmed by real-life experiences [12, 61–63]. In addition, the clinical assessment of CSU activity was not always uniform in all studies and different patient-reported outcome measures are used, either alone or in combination, to assess disease activity and guide the assessment of treatment efficacy.

Real-world studies have shown a response to treatment in 48–80% cases, while 7–14% are non-responders and 8–50% relapse after drug discontinuation [12, 55–61], supporting the efficacy and safety of omalizumab in CSU patients with an inadequate response to H1-antihistamines. These studies add precious information for the clinical management of CSU, but often present a relatively small sample size population and sometimes include different doses and administration timing of omalizumab. In particular, real-world studies demonstrated that omalizumab administration reduces the use of other CIndU/CSU-related medications. A recent large real-world retrospective study including 1546 patients with CIndU/CSU treated with omalizumab revealed that the majority started with a dosage of 300 mg and received the drug for an average of 9 months without dosing titration up or down [64]. Moreover, the use of other medications, such as corticosteroids and antidepressants, was consistently decreasing during the follow-up period, from 72.8% over the first 3 months to 58.5% over the last 3 months.

Additionally, real-life experiences have confirmed that there are different patient profiles according to omalizumab response [63, 65, 66]:

- patients typically show a response to treatment within the first 4–8 weeks (often within 1 week);
- patients initially non-responders can obtain a significant reduction in disease activity and even achieve "good control" (UAS7 ≤ 6) or "complete control" (UAS7 = 0) if the treatment is continued for up to 24 weeks.

Other different strategies mainly involve either modification of the omalizumab dose or a change in the treatment interval. Dose increases or reductions, if the complete CU symptoms control is achieved, should be stepwise [63].

Data on the response rate to omalizumab is available from meta-analyses and real-world evidence, but not all of them have assessed the time to response and, due to the different dosages and treatment durations, it is difficult to draw a common conclusion from these studies [32, 46, 49, 50, 53, 56, 57, 66–74]. Consequently, several parameters have been suggested to potentially predict treatment response, or possible treatment relapse. Some studies have been focused on different baseline clinical and laboratory parameters in order to identify the predictors of response to omalizumab in CSU patients. Asero et al. found that high levels of D-dimer seems to be a marker of response to treatment [32], but more recently the same authors and other studies indicate D-dimer only as a activity/severity marker in CSU patients and its plasma levels are reduced by omalizumab both in patients with and without angioedema at baseline [75]. Instead, many studies have shown that total IgE levels can be a marker of response to omalizumab [76]. Marzano et al. recently confirmed IgE basal levels as a reliable biomarker predicting response to treatment in CSU patients, while they did not support the usefulness of D-dimer [62]. In a single-center study on 47 CSU patients the baseline basophil FcεRI expression was found to be a potential immunological predictor of good and fast response to omalizumab (100% sensitivity and 73.2% specificity) [34].

The analysis of omalizumab responders in a prospective study of 64 patients showed that most basophil histamine release assay (BHRA)-positive patients responded only after the second injection, with a median time to response of 29 days, whereas BHRA-negative patients had a median time to response of only 2 days [77].

In a retrospective study of 41 antihistamine-refractory CU patients, the lack of basophil CD203c-upregulating activity in their serum correlated negatively with a clinical respond to omalizumab [78]. In detail, a significant association was found between the response and CD203c-upregulating activity, autoimmune phenotype, low IgE levels, and high eosinophil count levels.

Greater number of prior medications was associated with a lack of response to omalizumab in a study of 52 patients with severe CU, whereas the presence of anaphylaxis, angioedema, dermatographism, steroid use, and disease duration were not [79].

Furthermore, CSU duration before omalizumab and baseline UAS7 may be considered a negative markers of response and high relapse risk [62]. Although the response to omalizumab should not be dose dependent in CSU, real-life settings have shown that body mass index could influence the performance of the drug [17].

In a cohort of 154 patients the following factors were described as possible predictors of a favourable response to omalizumab [80]:

- diagnosis of CSU vs. CIndU;
- no prior treatment with immunosuppressant drugs;
- older age;
- shorter duration of symptoms;
- absence of angioedema;
- negative histamine release test.

Over 85% of patients who present these characteristics achieved a complete respond to treatment.

In relation to the dosing, the proportion of patients who showed complete response to omalizumab 150 mg ranged from 15–22% in clinical trials and from 36–79% in real-world studies. Regarding omalizumab 300 mg, the proportion of complete responders ranged from 34–44% in clinical trials and from 40% to 84.6% in real-life settings. However, not all real-world studies provided information on treatment duration. In few real-world studies where patients have received either/both omalizumab 150 mg and 300 mg, the complete response was observed in 47–83%. In addition, a complete response was achieved as early as the day after the administration of the first dose or within 5 months [66–74].

Real-world settings support that repeated treatment cycles should be required in several CSU patients [12, 70, 74, 81, 82]. Regarding the retreatment, omalizumab seems to be highly efficient in relapsed patients who previously had responded well [74]. An Italian retrospective clinical analysis revealed that the second cycle treatment with omalizumab is effective more quickly compared to the first cycle response [12]. Based on current international guidelines, omalizumab labelling information and experience in clinical practice, an Italian group provided treatment recommendations regarding the use of omalizumab in patients with CSU concluding that repeated cycles or extended treatment may be necessary in patients with disease relapse or late treatment response [81]. These authors suggested to continue the treatment when patients have a UAS7 > 6 and/or UCT < 12.

Among responders, after discontinuation of omalizumab the treatment can be resumed at a later stage with the same degree of symptom control [82].

All the real-world studies underlined the high safety prophile of omalizumab also in continuous and long-term administration. Finally, in a meta-analysis of 67 published reports, benefits and safety of omalizumab in the real-world treatment of CSU have met or exceeded results achieved in clinical trials [83].

3.3 Omalizumab performances optimization in clinical practice

Current evidence indicates that CSU usually last from 3 to 12 months, but patients may be affected for more than 1 year (sometimes even more than 5 years) [84]. However, recommendations regarding treatment duration and re-treatment after symptoms return are lacking. Nevertheless, the primary results of the OPTIMA study have shown that approximately 88% of patients who relapsed after being previously well-controlled with omalizumab, regain symptom control upon re-treatment within 3 months [85]. Similarly, phase IV XTEND-CIU study and few real-world studies have shown re-treatment to be effective in CSU patients who had previously responded to omalizumab but who relapsed after treatment withdrawal [4, 86]. To date, there are limited data comparing the therapeutic effect of omalizumab for patients with CSU, CIndU, and CSU plus CIndU. A recent chinese study revealed that omalizumab is highly effective and safe in 138 patients with difficult-to-treat CSU, CIndU, or both [87]. Among the CU patients enrolled, 87% responded to omalizumab therapy and those with higher baseline total IgE levels and longer disease durations showed more likely to experience rapid relapse after discontinuation of the drug.

Many other important questions regarding the use of omalizumab remain to be answered in order to optimize treatment management and patient outcomes. In particular, further investigations regarding predictors of good outcome, optimal dose, and dosing intervals based on treatment response to omalizumab in CSU are needed. A personalized therapeutic algorithm according to the patient clinical and bio-markers, modulated on the dose–response pattern, should facilitate the clinical management of omalizumab and help clinicians to determine the most appropriate therapeutic strategy for CSU. Future research is, therefore, required to evaluate the role of omalizumab in the various subtypes of CU as well as to establish standardized protocols for dosing and monitoring adverse effects of long-term therapy.

4. Ligelizumab (QGE031)

Even though omalizumab has been changing the management of CU, there is still a need for new targets and new biologics targeting new pathways in the management of the disease, which should provide long-lasting remission, be administered orally and cheaper. Among the CSU treatments that are still under clinical trials, there is anothers anti-IgE drug called ligelizumab (QGE031), which has been developed with the intention of overcoming some of the limitations associated with omalizumab [88].

4.1 Ligelizumab: what is it and how does it work in Chronic Spontaneous Urticaria

Ligelizumab, a next-generation high-affinity fully human monoclonal IgG anti-IgE antibody, demonstrated dose- and time-dependent suppression of free IgE, basophil FcεRI and basophil surface IgE superior in extent (free IgE and surface

IgE) and duration to omalizumab (**Table 1**) [89, 90]. Ligelizumab recognizes a distinct IgE epitope only partially overlapping with that of omalizumab, interacting across the IgE-Fc dimer and favors the recognition of IgE in an open conformation different from its FcεRI- or CD23-bound conformations. Moreover, it binds IgE with significantly higher affinity (almost 50-fold higher) than omalizumab and shows a correspondingly enhanced inhibition of IgE binding to FcεRI and basophil activation. However, ligelizumab is inferior to omalizumab in preventing IgE binding to CD23. Structural analysis indicates that differences in the ligelizumab epitope and spatial orientation on IgE contribute to this differential inhibition [91].

Indeed, ligelizumab and omalizumab recognize distinct binding epitopes in the IgE Cε3 domain, showing some overlap but also different sensitivities to IgE conformation. On one side, the increased affinity of ligelizumab for IgE is superior than omalizumab regarding neutralization of free serum IgE, on the other side the additional mode of action for ligelizumab through the inhibition of IgE production may provide additional therapeutic benefit. Indeed, ligelizumab is more efficient in suppressing FcεRI-dependent allergic reactions in an in vivo model, while omalizumab may have advantages in blocking antigen presentation and transport processes that are dependent on IgE:CD23 interactions [92, 93].

4.2 Ligelizumab clinical studies

Currently, ligelizumab is being developed solely for the treatment of CSU. Phase IIb randomized controlled trial (NCT02477332) in CSU (CQGE031C2201) results demonstrated ligelizumab to be efficacious at 72 mg and 240 mg dosage, showing superiority over omalizumab and a comparable good safety profile [94]. The subsequent extension study (NCT02649218) in CSU (CQGE031C2201E1) proved the efficacy and safety of the ligelizumab at the dose of 240 mg every 4 weeks for a 1-year period, achiving more prolonged symptom control compared to the core study [95, 96].

4.2.1 CQGE031C2201

This was a 20-weeks multi-center, randomized, double-blind, placebo- and active controlled phase IIb dose-range finding study in subjects with CSU inadequately controlled [94]. CSU patients included in the study had to have a moderate-to-severe CSU defined as UAS7 of at least 16, 7 days hives severity score (HSS7) of at least 8, and in-clinic UAS of at least 4 (range 1 to 6) on at least one of the screening visit days. Exclusion criteria were represented by a previous exposure to omalizumab or ligelizumab, any other skin disease that is associated with chronic itching that might confound the trial evaluations and results, and a clearly defined underlying cause of CU other than CSU (e.g., inducible urticaria).

Subjects were randomized into 1 of 6 parallel treatment arms at a ratio of 1:2:2:2:1:1 (subcutaneous injections every 4 weeks of ligelizumab 24 mg, 72 mg, or 240 mg, omalizumab at a dose of 300 mg, a single dose of ligelizumab 120 mg followed by placebo or placebo) for the 20-week treatment period. The single 120 mg dose of ligelizumab was used to gain blinded wash-out information in relation to return of symptoms.

During the screening, treatment, and follow-up periods, nonsedating H1-antihistamines were used as rescue medication. Moreover, as background medication, this trial required concurrent use of H1-antihistamines at locally approved doses or at increased doses up to four times alone or in combination with H2-antihistamines or leukotriene-receptor antagonists (montelukast, zafirlukast, or pranlukast), according to the EAACI/GA²LEN/EDF/WAO urticaria guideline at that time [1].

Primary end-point was the achievement of complete hives response (HSS7 = 0) at week 12 (four weeks after the last injection), similar to phase III trials of omalizumab. Among 574 patients screened, 382 were included and 338 completed the treatment phase. The mean age ± SD of the study population was 43.3 ± 12.5 years (range 18 to 75 years) and 75% of subjects were female. Mean time since diagnosis of CSU was 4.3 ± 6.0 years. Median IgE levels at baseline was 87.2 IU/ml (range 0 to 14100).

With ligelizumab the main objective of the trial was achieved, showing a dose–response relationship with respect to the achievement of a HSS7 of 0 at week 12. The relationship resulted in a plateau starting close to the 72 mg dose of ligelizumab, while no further improvement in response was noted with the dosage of 240 mg.

At week 12, complete hive response was achieved in 30%, 51%, and 42% of patients treated with 24 mg, 72 mg, and 240 mg ligelizumab, respectively. Instead, a HSS7 of 0 was achieved only in 26% of patients with omalizumab and in none of those in the placebo group. The 7 days itch severity score (ISS7) showed a pattern similar to that seen with the hives-severity score. At week 12, UAS7 of 0 was achieved in 30%, 44%, and 40% of patients treated with ligelizumab 24 mg, 72 mg, and 240 mg, respectively, in comparison to 26% with omalizumab and none with placebo. Considering the scores (ISS7, UAS7, and HSS7) achieved, ligelizumab demonstrated superiority not only over placebo but also over omalizumab. In addition to hives and itch the AAS decreased to −21.1, −37.6, and − 27.3 among patients treated with 24 mg, 72 mg, and 240 mg ligelizumab, respectively, in comparison to −23.1 in patients with omalizumab and − 23.6 in the placebo group.

At week 4, the effect of the single 120 mg ligelizumab dose was similar to that seen with 72 mg and 240 mg and lasted until week 8. In contrast, a partial relapse of symptoms was noted with the 72 mg ligelizumab toward the end of the administration interval of four weeks. These data gave evidence that a dose higher than 72 mg ligelizumab could potentially provide enough drug effect throughout the administration interval of four weeks, minimizing symptom relapse. In support of this sustained treatment effect, the median time to loss of complete response in patients who had an UAS7 of 0 at the end of the treatment (week 20) was greatest in the patients treated with 240 mg of ligelizumab (10.5 weeks), while was similar in the groups that received 72 mg of ligelizumab or 300 mg of omalizumab (4 weeks).

Similar to omalizumab, the most frequent AEs were mild to moderate injection site reactions after subcutaneous administration (4% and 7% of patients treated with the 72 mg and 240 mg, respectively). All other minor AEs (mainly upper respiratory infections and headaches) showed no meaningful difference among the trial groups. Deaths, anaphylaxis or serious adverse events to ligelizumab have not been reported.

4.2.2 CQGE031C2201E1

Patients who completed CQGE031C2201 were eligible to be enrolled in this extension study at week 32 that confirmed the safety of the long-term (52 weeks) administration of the highest dose of ligelizumab (subcutaneous injections every 4 weeks of ligelizumab 240 mg) [95]. At week 52, 61.1% of patients achieved UAS7 ≤ 6 and, after stopping treatment, the median time of well-controlled disease was 28.0 weeks. These results implicate a longer treatment effect of ligelizumab compared to omalizumab [96].

4.2.3 CQGE031C1301

CQGE031C1301 represents a phase II multi-center, open-label study (NCT03907878) to investigate the safety/tolerability and efficacy of ligelizumab

120 mg every 4 weeks in adult Japanese patients with CSU inadequately controlled with H1-antihistamines. Currently, CQGE031C1301 is still ongoing.

4.2.4 Phase III ligelizumab study

Currently, two similar trials (PEARL 1 NCT03580356 and PEARL 2 NCT03580369) are ongoing to study the efficacy and safety of ligelizumab (72 mg or 120 mg every 4 weeks) in CSU patients who remain symptomatic despite standard of care treatment [97]. Both are 52-weeks multi-center, randomized, double-blind, placebo- and active controlled phase III trials and is planned to enroll about 1000 patients for each study.

In addition, a phase IIIb extension study is planned to investigate ligelizumab in adult and adolescent patients with CSU (NCT04210843) [98].

Results from these studies may confirm whether ligelizumab should become an alternative first-line treatment option in H1-antihistamine refractory CSU patients.

5. Anti-IgE antibodies in Chronic Spontaneous Urticaria special populations and drug interactions

To date, ligelizumab have not been investigated pregnant women, children, elderly, history of cancer, patients with renal or hepatic impairment, while only few studies were published regarding the use omalizumab in these special populations.

5.1 Pregnancy

Currently, omalizumab is not approved for use in pregnancy and there are only few case reports published in literature describing omalizumab as an effective and safe therapy for urticaria in pregnant women [99–102].

The EXPECT study examined 250 women with with moderate-to-severe asthma exposed to omalizumab during pregnancy [102]. Each enrolled patient received at least one dose of omalizumab during pregnancy up to 8 weeks prior to conception. This study compared EXPECT outcomes with those from a disease-matched external population of pregnant women with moderate-to-severe asthma not treated with omalizumab. No significant difference in spontaneous abortions, major congenital anomalies, prematurity, or low birth weight was observed among pregnant women exposed to omalizumab compared with the disease-matched unexposed cohort. However, given the observational nature of this registry, an absence of increased risk with omalizumab cannot be definitively established. Therefore, omalizumab might be considered in pregnant women, but to date its use during pregnancy is not recommended by any accepted international or national guideline. Randomized controlled trials should be conducted on omalizumab during pregnancy before complete reassurance of the drug is established.

5.2 Children

Randomized controlled trials using omalizumab in urticaria included only a small number of 39 adolescent patients (aged ≥12 years) [103]. Passanisi et al. reported a case series of six children (66.7% males) with a mean age of 14.7 years (range 11–16 years) treated with at least one 6-months course of omalizumab [103]. The average follow-up period was 13 ± 6 months and only one patient was no responder, while three patients needed a second course of treatment. This study demonstrated that omalizumab is effective and safe as treatment option for CSU unresponsive adolescent patients. Moreover, Passanisi et al. summarized in his study the 12 previously published case reports. Applied omalizumab doses ranged from 75 mg every 4 weeks to 300 mg every 2 weeks for a period of up to 12 months, but most patients received the standard dose of 300 mg every 4 weeks.

Recently, a retrospective multi-center case series reported the use of omalizumab in 19 children (6 to 16.9 years old) with recalcitrant CSU [104]. Sixteen (84%) responded to omalizumab, although two became non-responsive after 6–12 months of therapy, while three patients (16%) were resistant to treatment, achieving remission through fourth-line (Cyclosporine A) or other therapies. This study stated that children with recalcitrant CSU, even those <12 years old, respond well to standard-dose of omalizumab at rates similar to adults. Future prospective randomized clinical trials of omalizumab and other anti-IgE therapies in children are needed.

5.3 Elderly (65 Years and Older)

Whilst the randomized clinical trials had an upper age limit of 75 years, the mean age of all included CSU patients was within the range of 40–45 years. Therefore, limited data are now available on the use of anti-IgE antibodies in patients older than 65 years, but there is no evidence that elderly patients require a different dose from younger adult patients. A recent Italian real-life experience on 32 patients ≥65 years of age found that omalizumab is a well-tolerated and effective therapy for elderly patients with nonsedating H1-antihistamine-refractory CSU [105].

5.4 History of cancer

To date, there are only few reports of effective and safe omalizumab treatment in patients with a history of previous cancer (e.g. with breast carcinoma, in-situ melanoma, thyroid carcinoma, laryngeal carcinoma, and pituitary adenoma) [106], while evidence in patients with active malignant disease is scarce. Very rarely CU can be caused by cancer and if so, resolves with its cure [107]. Therefore, current expert opinion suggested that omalizumab can be used in patients with cancer [108].

5.5 Patients with renal or hepatic impairment

As IgG monoclonal antibodies are mainly eliminated via intracellular catabolism, renal impairment or hepatic impairment is not expected to influence clearance of ligelizumab and omalizumab. No dedicated drug–drug interaction studies have been conducted so far. Hepatic metabolizing enzymes are not involved in monoclonal antibody elimination, consequentely no pharmacokinetic interactions with co-administered medicinal products are expected with the both medications.

6. The future in Chronic Spontaneous Urticaria: anti-IgE antibodies and beyond

In addition to drug repurposing as in anti-IL-4/13, IL-5, and IL-17 antibodies, novel targeted therapy options are currently undergoing clinical trials and will be available in the near future: other anti-IgE antibodies such as UB-221 and Quilizumab, molecules targeting intracellular signaling pathways such as spleen tyrosine kinase inhibitors, surface inhibitory molecules such as siglec-8, anti-IL-1s such as canakinumab, Bruton kinase inhibitors such as GDC-0853 and anti-IL-5s such as benralizumab and mepolizumab [5, 109]. New potential target molecules are going to be proposed as novel treatments and have been rapidly developing.

6.1 UB-221

UB-221 is a humanized IgG1 mAb (clone 8D6) that targets the Cε3 domain of IgE antibody and, unlike omalizumab, it can bind to IgE bound by CD23 (**Table 1**). UB-221 neutralizes IgE without activation of mast cells and basophils and was superior to omalizumab while targeting IgE by 3- to 8-folds in terms of pharmacologic effects. It is currently being investigated in two ongoing phase I trials for safety, tolerability, pharmacodynamics, and pharmacokinetics following a single dose (0.2, 0.6, 2, 6, 10 mg/kg UB-221 intravenously vs. placebo) in adult patients with CSU inadequately controlled with H1-antihistamines (NCT03632291 in Taiwan, and NCT04175704, location not provided).

6.2 Quilizumab

Quilizumab is a humanized, afucosylated, monoclonal IgG1 antibody, that binds membrane-bound IgE on B cells at the M1-prime segment, which is absent in soluble IgE (**Table 1**). In healthy volunteers and patients with allergic rhinitis or asthma, this anti-IgE antibody resulted able to reduce the total and specific IgE serum levels for at least 6 months after the last dose [110, 111]. This may implicate that quilizumab affects long-term IgE memory and bears the capacity for a sustained effect compared to omalizumab. Regarding quilizumab, there is no published evidence about its effect on angioedema and only one clinical trial is currently ongoing (NCT01987947) in CU. A previous randomized trial of quilizumab in adults with refractory CSU revealed that, although it reduced median serum IgE levels by approximately 30% over 20 weeks, it did not cause clinically relevant effects as assessed by ISS7 and UAS7 [112]. The study investigators hypothesized that the remaining serum IgE may be produced by long-lived IgE plasma cells that are not targeted by the drug due to their lack of membrane IgE.

6.3 Other possible targets for treatment

Some other molecules participating in the pathogenesis of CSU might be important targets for treatment in the upcoming years.

- In patients with CSU, C5a has been shown to enhance histamine release from mast cells upon activation of FcεRI through IgG autoantibodies [113]. Moreover, activation with C5a led to an increased basophil response in patients with CU compared to healthy controls [114]. These finding indicate a possible role for C5a in CSU and provide a basis for the evaluation of C5a inhibitors (IFX-1, eculizumab) in the treatment of CSU [115].

- SHIP has been shown to be a key "gatekeeper" of mast cell degranulation. [116]. Indeed, SHIP acts as a negative regulator of degranulation by hydrolyzing phosphatidylinositol-3,4,5-trisphosphate, a second messenger generated in activated cells by phosphatidylinositol 3-kinase. SHIP-negative mast cells are more likely to degranulate following IgE binding. Instead, CD200R represents a novel and potent inhibitory receptor that can be targeted in vivo to regulate mast cell-dependent pathologies [117]. Considering their regulatory functions on mast cells, the use of SHIP and CD200R antibodies might be of interest in CSU.

- Histamine H4 receptors (H4R) are expressed by hematopoietic cells including eosinophils, mast cells, neutrophils, and T cells. Activation of H4 receptors results in chemotaxis, cytokine production, immunomodulation, and inflammatory cell trafficking [118]. The use of H4R-antagonist called JNJ-7777120 has been associated with reduction of histamine-mediated scratching and Th2-induced inflammation in dermatitis [119]. Another H4R-antagonist, ZPL-3893787, improve inflammatory skin lesions in patients with atopic dermatitis compared to placebo [120]. The anti-inflammatory and anti-pruritic effects of H4R-antagonists might be of benefit in CSU treatment.

- IL-31 is a pro-inflammatory cytokine mainly secreted by Th2 cells that exerts its effects through two receptors: IL-31 receptor A and oncostatin M receptor (OSMR) [121]. Increased expression of OSMR protein and histamine release were also shown in chronic autoimmune urticaria. In addition, OSMR gene silencing in mice led to a decrease in inflammatory cytokines and number of eosinophils [122]. These data indicate that IL-31 or OSMRβ inhibitors (e.g., nemolizumab, vixarelimab) might play an interesting role in the treatment of CSU.

- Increased levels of IL-6, another pro-inflammatory cytokine, have been demonstrated in patients with CSU [123]. It was also correlated with disease severity, suggesting the role of systemic inflammation in CSU. Tocilizumab, an IL-6 monoclonal antibody, led to improvement in patients with Schnitzler syndrome, and might be of potential benefit for CSU treatment [124].

- The increased expression of Mas-related gene X2, which is a receptor for histamine-releasing neuropeptides including substance P and vasoactive intestinal peptides, was demonstrated to be a possible therapeutic target in mast cells of patients with CSU [125].

- The antagonists for neurokinin receptor-1 (e.g., aprepitant, tradipitant), which is the main cutaneous receptor for substance P, are under investigation for atopic dermatitis for their antipruritic effects and they might be of value for CSU as well [126].

- The expression of thymic stromal lymphopoietin (TSLP), a promotor of Th2 response, was shown to be increased in patients with CSU, thus making the anti-TSLP monoclonal antibody, tezepelumab, a potential treatment option for CSU [127].

- Calcium Release-Activated Calcium Modulator 1 (CRACM1/ORAI1) is a subtype of Ca2+ membrane channel, causing Ca2+ influx into the cells and mast cell degranulation [128]. Ca2+ is an essential element that regulates immune responses, especially in the development and function of T and B cells, and therefore ORAI1 is considered to participate in allergic diseases. Jie et al. have demonstrated that different single nucleotide polymorphisms in the ORAI1 gene are associated with an increased risk of CSU and better response to desloratadine [129]. Thus, targeting of ORAI1 via silencing RNAs might be of therapeutic value in CSU.

7. Conclusions

The introduction of anti-IgE antibodies in urticaria management has been representing a milestone in the treatment of H1-antihistamine refractory patients.

Name of the Study	Phase	Indication	Patients included	Anti-IgE antibodies dose every 4 weeks	Efficacy on Angioedema	Outcome with anti-IgE antibodies	Outcome with placebo	Year of publication [reference]
X-CUISITE	II	Chronic spontaneous urticaria° (patients exhibit IgE against thyroperoxidase)	49	• Omalizumab 75 to 375 mg according to baseline IgE and body weight	Not evaluated with score	*Week 24* UAS7 = −17.8 DLQI = −6.3 CU-Q2oL = −21	*Week 24* UAS7 = −7.9 DLQI = −1.5 CU-Q2oL = −2.3	2011 [50]
MYSTIQUE	II	Chronic spontaneous urticaria°	90	• A single dose of omalizumab 75 mg • A single dose of omalizumab 300 mg • A single dose of omalizumab 600 mg	—	*Week 4* • Omalizumab 75 mg UAS7 = −9.8 ISS7 = −4.5 HSS7 = −5.3 • Omalizumab 300 mg UAS7 = −19.9 ISS7 = −9.2 HSS7 = −10.7 • Omalizumab 600 mg UAS7 = −14.6 ISS7 = −6.5 HSS7 = −8.1	*Week 4* UAS7 = −6.9 ISS7 = −3.5 HSS7 = −3.5	2011 [49]
MoA	II	Chronic spontaneous urticaria° (healthy controls included)	40	• Omalizumab 300 mg	AEFD	*Week 4 to 12* AEFD = 90.9 *Week 12* UAS7 = −23.1 CUQ2oL = −39.2 DLQI = −10.2	*Week 4 to 12* AEFD = 70.5 *Week 12* UAS7 = −8.1 CUQ2oL = −5.7 DLQI = −3.1	2019 [130]

Name of the Study	Phase	Indication	Patients included	Anti-IgE antibodies dose every 4 weeks	Efficacy on Angioedema	Outcome with anti-IgE antibodies	Outcome with placebo	Year of publication [reference]
X-ACT	III	Chronic spontaneous urticaria°	91	• Omalizumab 300 mg	AEBD AE-QoL MAEBD MTFRAE	*Week 0 to 28* AEBD = 14.6 MAEBD = 9 days *Week 28* UAS7 = −16.8 CUQ2oL = −30.9 DLQI = −10.5 AE-QoL = −41.4 MTFRAE = 56–63 days	*Week 0 to 28* AEBD = 49.5 MAEBD = 30 days *Week 28* UAS7 = −6.5 CUQ2oL = −12.1 DLQI = −5.6 AE-QoL = −24.2 MTFRAE = <5 days	2016, 2018 [131, 132]
ASTERIA I	III	Chronic spontaneous urticaria°	319	• Omalizumab 75 mg • Omalizumab 150 mg • Omalizumab 300 mg	AEFD	*Week 4 to 12* • Omalizumab 75 mg AEFD = 86.5 • Omalizumab 150 mg AEFD = 89.6 • Omalizumab 300 mg AEFD = 96.1 *Week 12* • Omalizumab 75 mg UAS7 = −13.8 ISS7 = −6.5 HSS7 = −7.4 DLQI = −6.3 CU-Q2oL = −19.2 • Omalizumab 150 mg UAS7 = −14.4 ISS7 = −6.7 HSS7 = −7.8 DLQI = −8.0 CU-Q2oL = −23.1 • Omalizumab 300 mg UAS7 = −20.8	*Week 4 to 12* AEFD = 88.2 *Week 12* UAS7 = −8.0 ISS7 = −3.6 HSS7 = −4.4 DLQI = −6.1 CU-Q2oL = −19.7 *Week 24* UAS7 = −11.73 ISS7 = −5.4 HSS7 = −6.3 *Week 40 (at the end of 16 weeks of follow-up)* DLQI = −7.9	2015 [54]

Name of the Study	Phase	Indication	Patients included	Anti-IgE antibodies dose every 4 weeks	Efficacy on Angioedema	Outcome with anti-IgE antibodies	Outcome with placebo	Year of publication [reference]
						ISS7 = −9.4 HSS7 = −11.4 DLQI = −10.3 CU-Q2oL = −30.5 *Week 24* • Omalizumab 75 mg UAS7 = −14.9 ISS7 = −7.0 HSS7 = −8.0 • Omalizumab 150 mg UAS7 = −14.2 ISS7 = −6.5 HSS7 = −7.8 • Omalizumab 300 mg UAS7 = −22.1 ISS7 = −9.8 HSS7 = −12.3 *Week 40 (at the end of 16 weeks of follow-up)* • Omalizumab 75 mg DLQI = −7.0 • Omalizumab 150 mg DLQI = −5.2 • Omalizumab 300 mg DLQI = −4.9		
ASTERIA II	III	Chronic spontaneous urticaria°	323	• Omalizumab 75 mg • Omalizumab 150 mg • Omalizumab 300 mg	AEFD	*Week 4 to 12* • Omalizumab 75 mg AEFD = 93.5 • Omalizumab 150 mg AEFD = 91.6 • Omalizumab 300 mg	*Week 4 to 12* AEFD = 89.2 *Week 12* UAS7 = −10.4 ISS7 = −5.1 HSS7 = −5.2	2013 [52]

Name of the Study	Phase	Indication	Patients included	Anti-IgE antibodies dose every 4 weeks	Efficacy on Angioedema	Outcome with anti-IgE antibodies	Outcome with placebo	Year of publication [reference]
						AEFD = 95.5 *Week 12* • Omalizumab 75 mg UAS7 = −13.82 ISS7 = −5.9 HSS7 = −7.2 DLQI = −7.5 CU-Q2oL = −20.6 • Omalizumab 150 mg UAS7 = −17.9 ISS7 = −8.1 HSS7 = −9.8 DLQI = −8.3 CU-Q2oL = −27.0 • Omalizumab 300 mg UAS7 = −21.7 ISS7 = −9.8 HSS7 = −12.0 DLQI = −10.2 CU-Q2oL = −31.4	DLQI = −6.1 CU-Q2oL = −17.7	
GLACIAL	III	Chronic spontaneous urticaria*	336	• Omalizumab 300 mg	AEFD	*Week 4 to 12* AEFD = 91.0 *Week 12* UAS7 = −19.0 ISS7 = −8.6 HSS7 = −10.5 DLQI = −9.7 CU-Q2oL = −29.3	*Week 4 to 12* AEFD = 88.1 *Week 12* UAS7 = −8.5 ISS7 = −4.6 HSS7 = −4.5 DLQI = −5.1 CU-Q2oL = −16.3	2013 [53]

Name of the Study	Phase	Indication	Patients included	Anti-IgE antibodies dose every 4 weeks	Efficacy on Angioedema	Outcome with anti-IgE antibodies	Outcome with placebo	Year of publication [reference]
POLARIS	III	Chronic spontaneous urticaria°	218	• Omalizumab 150 mg • Omalizumab 300 mg	—	*Week 12* • Omalizumab 150 mg UAS7 = −18.8 ISS7 = −8.8 HSS7 = −10.0 DLQI = −7.2 • Omalizumab 300 mg UAS7 = −22.4 ISS7 = −10.2 HSS7 = −12.2 DLQI = −8.4	*Week 12* UAS7 = −13.9 ISS7 = −6.5 HSS7 = −7.4 DLQI = −5.3	2018 [133]
UFO	II	Symptomatic dermographism	61	• Omalizumab 150 mg • Omalizumab 300 mg	—	*Week 10* • Omalizumab 150 mg CFT = −1.8 CR = 44% • Omalizumab 300 mg CFT = −2.0 CR = 53%	*Week 10* CFT = −0.6 CR = 11%	2017 [134]
CUN-OMAL-UCOL	II	Cholinergic urticaria§	22	• Omalizumab 300 mg (first 4 months blinded, followed by 8 months open-label)	—	*Week 16* No difference in negative exercise challenge test rate compared to placebo UCOL score = −28 CU-Q2oL = −7.6 VAS = −10 *Week 48* Negative exercise challenge test: 31% Significant progressive improvement along time starting from week 16	*Week 16* UCOL score = −16 CU-Q2oL = −6.5 VAS = −10 *Week 48* Theoretical negative exercise challenge test: 11%	2019 [135]

Name of the Study	Phase	Indication	Patients included	Anti-IgE antibodies dose every 4 weeks	Efficacy on Angioedema	Outcome with anti-IgE antibodies	Outcome with placebo	Year of publication [reference]
CUTEX	II	Cold urticaria	31	• Omalizumab 150 mg • Omalizumab 300 mg	—	*Week 10* • Omalizumab 150 mg CTT = −10.6°C CR = 40% • Omalizumab 300 mg CTT = −10.4°C CR = 44%	*Week 10* CTT = −0.3°C CR = 0%	2017 [136]
XOLUS	II	Solar urticaria	10	• Omalizumab 300 mg	—	*Week 12* MUDi = 20% DLQI <6 = 40% VAS50 = 40% *Week 20* MUDi = 0% DLQI <6 = 11% VAS50 = 0%	No placebo arm; comparison to baseline	2016 [137]
CQGE031C2201	IIb	Chronic spontaneous urticaria*	382	• Ligelizumab 24 mg • Ligelizumab 72 mg • Ligelizumab 240 mg • Omalizumab 300 mg	AAS7	*Week 12* • Ligelizumab 24 mg UAS7 = −16.0 ISS7 = −7.0 HSS7 = −9.0 AAS7 = −20.0 • Ligelizumab 72 mg UAS7 = −27.0 ISS7 = −10.3 HSS7 = −16.5 AAS7 = −37.6 • Ligelizumab 240 mg	*Week 12* UAS7 = −13.0 ISS7 = −5.0 HSS7 = −7.5 AAS7 = −23.6 *Week 20* UAS7 = −12.0 ISS7 = −5.5 HSS7 = −6.5 AAS7 = −24.4	2019 [94]

Name of the Study	Phase	Indication	Patients included	Anti-IgE antibodies dose every 4 weeks	Efficacy on Angioedema	Outcome with anti-IgE antibodies	Outcome with placebo	Year of publication [reference]
						UAS7 = −22.9 ISS7 = −10.0 HSS7 = −14.0 AAS7 = −29.9 • Omalizumab 300 mg UAS7 = −18.5 ISS7 = −8.8 HSS7 = −11.0 AAS7 = −25.0 *Week 20* • Ligelizumab 24 mg UAS7 = −19.5 ISS7 = −7.5 HSS7 = −9.75 AAS7 = −22.6 • Ligelizumab 72 mg UAS7 = −26.5 ISS7 = −9.5 HSS7 = −15.5 AAS7 = −35.2 • Ligelizumab 240 mg UAS7 = −21.8 ISS7 = −9.0 HSS7 = −13.5 AAS7 = −27.3 • Omalizumab 300 mg UAS7 = −19.0 ISS7 = −8.0 HSS7 = −11.0 AAS7 = −23.1		

Name of the Study	Phase	Indication	Patients included	Anti-IgE antibodies dose every 4 weeks	Efficacy on Angioedema	Outcome with anti-IgE antibodies	Outcome with placebo	Year of publication [reference]
QUAIL	IIb	Chronic spontaneous urticaria^	32	• Quilizumab 450 mg	—	*Week 20* UAS7 = −2.0 ISS7 = −5.3 HSS7 = −0	*Week 20* UAS7 = −11.0 ISS7 = −2.2 HSS7 = −3.5	2016 [112]

Abbreviations: *7 days Angioedema Severity Score, AAS7; 7 days Hives-Severity Score, HSS7; 7 days Itch Severity Score, ISS7; 7 days Urticaria Activity Score, UAS7; Angioedema Free Days, AEFD; Angioedema Burdened Days, AEBD; Angioedema Quality of Life, AE-QoL; Cholinergic Urticaria score, UCOL score; Chronic Urticaria Quality of Life, CU-Q2oL; critical friction threshold, CFT; complete response, CR; Dermatology Life Quality Index, DLQI; Median Angioedema Burdened Days, MAEBD; Median Time to First Recurrence of Angioedema after last injection of study drug, MTFRAE; >10-fold increase in minimal urticarial dose, MUDi; Visual Analogue Scale, VAS; 50% improvement from baseline measured on a visual analog scale, VAS50.*
°*Inadequately controlled by H1-antihistamine at approved dose.*
§*Inadequately controlled with a doubled dose of H1-antihistamine.*
^*Inadequately controlled with H1-antihistamines at approved or increased doses alone or in combination with leukotriene receptor antagonists.*
**Inadequately controlled with H1-antihistamines at approved or increased doses alone or in combination with H2-antihistamines or leukotriene receptor antagonists.*

Table 2.
Clinical Efficacy of Anti-IgE Antibodies in Phase II and III randomised controlled trials of Chronic Urticaria.

The results of the anti-IgE antibodies on CU in phase II and III randomised controlled trials [49, 50, 53, 54, 94, 112, 130–137] were summarized in **Table 2**.

Omalizumab 300 mg every 4 weeks, as add-on therapy, has demonstrated effective and safe in most, but not all, patients with CSU and there is evidence that this holds true for angioedema and CIndU. However, additional studies, using registries, real life settings and controlled trials should investigate personalized dosages and administration intervals, based on e. g. body mass index, UAS7 results, and on the identification of biomarkers able to predict changes in disease activity in response to therapy, for the development of tailored treatment algorithms to be used in clinical practice.

Current data of ligelizumab, being the next-generation anti-IgE antibody that is one-step ahead in clinical trials, are very promising and it has the potential to be a valid alternative for CSU patients unresponsive to omalizumab. If the phase III trial program confirms the superiority of ligelizumab compared to omalizumab, there is hope that symptoms might be controlled in all patients with CSU.

There are no licensed treatment options for CIndU and, therefore, recommended treatment is similar to CSU. However, off-label use of omalizumab has shown to be less effective compared to in CSU. Results from randomized controlled trials of ligelizumab for CIndU seem to be highly encouraging.

It will be intersting to see whether next-generation anti-IgE therapies are effective in CSU, CIndU and angioedema. The mechanism of action of the various anti-IgE approaches should be further elucidated in order to optimize the treatment of CU patients and its better understanding might enable targeted therapy in the near future.

Acknowledgements

The chapter was funded by Novartis Farma S.p.A.

Author contributions

All authors made substantive intellectual contributions to the published chapter, and each author listed on the publication has seen and approved the submission of the chapter.

Funding

Honorarium, grant, or other form of payment was not given to anyone of the authors to produce the chapter.

Conflict of interest

The authors declare that they have no competing interests.

Nomenclature

AAS	Angioedema Activity Score.
AE-QoL	Angioedema Quality of Life.
AEs	Adverse Effects.

ASST	Autologous Serum Skin Test.
AU	Acute Urticaria.
BHRA	Basophil Histamine Release Assay.
CIndU	Chronic Inducible Urticaria.
CRACM1/ORAI1	Calcium Release-Activated Calcium Modulator 1.
CsA	Cyclosporine A.
CU	Chronic Urticaria.
CU-Q2oL	Chronic Urticaria Quality of Life.
CSU	Chronic Spontaneous Urticaria.
FcεRI	IgE Fc receptor.
H4R	Histamine H4 receptors.
HSS7	7 days Hives Severity Score.
Ig	Immunoglobulins.
IL	Interleukin.
ISS	Itch Severity Score.
ISS7	7 days Itch Severity Score.
OSMR	oncostatin M receptor.
QoL	Quality of Life.
TSLP	Thymic Stromal Lymphopoietin.
UAS	Urticaria Activity Score.
UAS7	7 days Urticaria Activity Score.
UCT	Urticaria Control Test.

Author details

Patrizia Pepe* and Victor Desmond Mandel
Dermatology Unit, Surgical, Medical and Dental Department of Morphological Sciences related to Transplant, Oncology and Regenerative Medicine, University of Modena and Reggio Emilia, Modena, Italy

*Address all correspondence to: patrizia.pepe@unimore.it

References

[1] Zuberier T, Aberer W, Asero R, et al. The EAACI/ GA2LEN/EDF/WAO guideline for the definition, classification, diagnosis and management of urticaria. Allergy. 2018; 73(7):1393–1414. DOI: 10.1111/all.13397

[2] Deacock SJ. An approach to the patient with urticaria. Clin Exp Immunol. 2008;153(2):151–161. DOI: 10.1111/j.1365-2249.2008.03693.x

[3] Antia C, Baquerizo K, Korman A, Bernstein JA, Alikhan A. Urticaria: A comprehensive review: Epidemiology, diagnosis, and work-up. J Am Acad Dermatol. 2018;79(4):599–614. DOI: 10.1016/j.jaad.2018.01.020

[4] Zuberbier T, Maurer M. Urticaria: current opinions about etiology, diagnosis and therapy. Acta Derm Venereol. 2007;87(3):196–205. DOI: 10.2340/00015555-0240

[5] Mandel VD, Alicandro T, Pepe P, et al. Chronic Spontaneous Urticaria: A Review of Pathological Mechanisms, Diagnosis, Clinical Management, and Treatment EMJ. 2020;5(1):29–39.

[6] Balp MM, Weller K, Carboni V, Chirilov A, Papavassilis C, Severin T. Prevalence and clinical characteristics of chronic spontaneous urticaria in pediatric patients. Pediatr Allergy Immunol. 2018;29(6):630–636. DOI: 10.1111/pai.12910

[7] O'Donnell BF, Lawlor F, Simpson J, Morgan M, Greaves MW. The impact of chronic urticaria on the quality of life. Br J Dermatol. 1997;136(2):197–201.

[8] Maurer M, Weller K, Bindslev-Jensen C, et al. Unmet clinical needs in chronic spontaneous urticaria. A GA^{2}LEN task force report. Allergy. 2011;66(3):317–330. DOI: 10.1111/j.1398-9995.2010.02496.x

[9] Gonçalo M, Gimenéz-Arnau A, Al-Ahmad M, et al. The global burden of chronic urticaria for the patient and society. Br J Dermatol. 2021;184(2):226–236. DOI: 10.1111/bjd.19561

[10] Weller K, Giménez-Arnau A, Grattan C, et al. The Chronic Urticaria Registry: rationale, methods and initial implementation. J Eur Acad Dermatol Venereol. 2020 Sep 18. DOI: 10.1111/jdv.16947

[11] Weller K, Groffik A, Magerl M, et al. Development, validation and initial results of the Angioedema Activity Score. Allergy. 2013;68(9):1185–1192. DOI: 10.1111/all.12209

[12] Mandel VD, Guanti MB, Liberati S, Demonte A, Pellacani P, Pepe P. Omalizumab in chronic spontaneous urticaria refractory to conventional therapy: an italian retrospective clinical analysis with suggestions for long-term maintenance strategies. Dermatol Ther (Heidelb). 2018;8(2):291–301. DOI: 10.1007/s13555-018-0240-7

[13] Kulthanan K, Chaweekulrat P, Komoltri C, et al. Cyclosporine for Chronic Spontaneous Urticaria: A Meta-Analysis and Systematic Review. J Allergy Clin Immunol Pract. 2018;6(2): 586–599. DOI: 10.1016/j.jaip.2017.07.017

[14] Grattan CE, O'Donnell BF, Francis DM, et al. Randomized double-blind study of cyclosporin in chronic "idiopathic" urticaria. Br J Dermatol. 2000;143(2):365–372. DOI: 10.1046/j.1365-2133.2000.03664.x

[15] Vena GA, Cassano N, Colombo D, Peruzzi E, Pigatto P, Neo-I-30 Study Group. Cyclosporine in chronic idiopathic urticaria: a double-blind, randomized, placebo-controlled trial J Am Acad Dermatol. 2006;55(4):705–709. DOI: 10.1016/j.jaad.2006.04.078

[16] Guillén-Aguinaga S, Jáuregui Presa I, Aguinaga-Ontoso E, Guillén-Grima F, Ferrer M. Updosing nonsedating antihistamines in patients with chronic spontaneous urticaria: a systematic review and meta-analysis. Br J Dermatol. 2016;175(6):1153–1165. DOI: 10.1111/bjd.14768

[17] Curto-Barredo L, Archilla LR, Vives GR, Pujol RM, Giménez-Arnau AM. Clinical Features of Chronic Spontaneous Urticaria that Predict Disease Prognosis and Refractoriness to Standard Treatment. Acta Derm Venereol. 2018;98(7):641–647. DOI: 10.2340/00015555-2941

[18] Chaplin DD. Overview of the immune response. J Allergy Clin Immunol. 2010;125(2 Suppl 2):S3–23. DOI: 10.1016/j.jaci.2009.12.980

[19] Schroeder HW Jr, Cavacini L. Structure and function of immunoglobulins. J Allergy Clin Immunol. 2010;125(2 Suppl 2):S41–S52. DOI: 10.1016/j.jaci.2009.09.046

[20] Amarasekera M. Immunoglobulin E in health and disease. Asia Pac Allergy. 2011;1(1):12–15. DOI: 10.5415/apallergy.2011.1.1.12

[21] Hu J, Chen J, Ye L, Cai Z, Sun J, Ki K. Anti-IgE therapy for IgE-mediated allergic diseases: from neutralizing IgE antibodies to eliminating IgE(+) B cells. Clin Transl Allergy. 2018;8:27. DOI: 10.1186/s13601-018-0213-z

[22] Wu LC, Zarrin AA. The production and regulation of IgE by the immune system. Nat Rev Immunol. 2014;14(4): 247–259. DOI: 10.1038/nri3632

[23] Ribatti D. The discovery of immunoglobulin E. Immunol Lett. 2016; 171:1–4. DOI: 10.1016/j.imlet.2016.01.001

[24] Dings RPM, Miller MC, Griffin RJ, Mayo KH. Galectins as Molecular Targets for Therapeutic Intervention. Int J Mol Sci. 2018;19(3):905. DOI: 10.3390/ijms19030905

[25] Kawakami T, Blank U. From IgE to Omalizumab. J Immunol. 2016;197(11): 4187–4192. DOI: 10.4049/jimmunol.1601476

[26] Johansson SG. The discovery of immunoglobulin e and its role in allergy. Chem Immunol Allergy. 2014;100:150–154. DOI: 10.1159/000358621

[27] Kaplan AP. Biologic agents in the treatment of urticaria. Curr Allergy Asthma Rep. 2012;12(4):288–291. DOI: 10.1007/s11882-012-0268-1

[28] Metz M, Staubach P, Bauer A, et al. Clinical efficacy of omalizumab in chronic spontaneous urticaria is associated with a reduction of FcεRI-positive cells in the skin. Theranostics. 2017;7(5):1266–1276. DOI: 10.7150/thno.18304

[29] Kaplan AP, Greaves M. Pathogenesis of chronic urticaria. Clin Exp Allergy. 2009;39(6):777–787. DOI: 10.1111/j.1365-2222.2009.03256.x

[30] Kaplan AP, Giménez-Arnau AM, Saini SS. Mechanisms of action that contribute to efficacy of omalizumab in chronic spontaneous urticaria. Allergy. 2017;72(4):519–533. DOI: 10.1111/all.13083

[31] Beck LA, Marcotte GV, MacGlashan D, Togias A, Saini S. Omalizumab-induced reductions in mast cell FcεRI expression and function. J Allergy Clin Immunol. 2004;114(3): 527–530. DOI: 10.1016/j.jaci.2004.06.032

[32] Asero R, Marzano AV, Ferrucci S, Cugno M. D-dimer plasma levels parallel the clinical response to omalizumab in patients with severe chronic spontaneous urticaria. Int Arch

Allergy Immunol. 2017;172(1):40–44. DOI: 10.1159/000453453

[33] Serrano-Candelas E, Martinez-Aranguren R, Valero A, et al. Comparable actions of omalizumab on mast cells and basophils. Clin Exp Allergy. 2016;46(1):92–102. DOI: 10.1111/cea.12668

[34] Deza G, Bertolín-Colilla M, Pujol RM, et al. Basophil FcεRI Expression in Chronic Spontaneous Urticaria: A Potential Immunological Predictor of Response to Omalizumab Therapy. Acta Derm Venereol. 2017;97 (6):698–704. DOI: 10.2340/00015555-2654

[35] Kolkhir P, Church MK, Weller K, Metz M, Schmetzer O, Maurer M. Autoimmune chronic spontaneous urticaria: what we know and what we do not know. *J Allergy Clin Immunol.* 2017; 139(6):1772–1781.e1. DOI: 10.1016/j.jaci.2016.08.050

[36] Bar-Sela S, Reshef T, Mekori YA. IgE antithyroid microsomal antibodies in a patient with chronic urticaria. J Allergy Clin Immunol. 1999;103(6): 1216–1217. DOI: 10.1016/s0091-6749 (99)70204-6

[37] Altrichter S, Peter HJ, Pisarevskaja D, Metz M, Martus P, Maurer M. IgE mediated autoallergy against thyroid peroxidase–a novel pathomechanism of chronic spontaneous urticaria? PLoS One. 2011;6 (4):e14794. DOI: 10.1371/journal.pone.0014794

[38] Kolkhir P, Metz M, Altrichter S, Maurer M. Comorbidity of chronic spontaneous urticaria and autoimmune thyroid diseases: A systematic review. Allergy. 2017;72(10):1440–1460. DOI: 10.1111/all.13182

[39] Cugno M, Asero R, Ferrucci S, et al. Elevated IgE to tissue factor and thyroglobulin are abated by omalizumab in chronic spontaneous urticaria. Allergy. 2018;73(12):2408–2411. DOI: 10.1111/all.13587

[40] Schmetzer O, Lakin E, Topal FA, et al. IL-24 is a common and specific autoantigen of IgE in patients with chronic spontaneous urticaria. J Allergy Clin Immunol. 2018;142(3):876–882. DOI: 10.1016/j.jaci.2017.10.035

[41] Hatada Y, Kashiwakura J, Hayama K, et al. Significantly high levels of anti-dsDNA immunoglobulin E in sera and the ability of dsDNA to induce the degranulation of basophils from chronic urticaria patients. Int Arch Allergy Immunol. 2013;161(Suppl 2): 154–158. DOI: 10.1159/000350388

[42] Gruber BL, Baeza ML, Marchese MJ, Agnello V, Kaplan AP. Prevalence and functional role of anti-IgE autoantibodies in urticarial syndromes. J Invest Dermatol. 1988;90(2):213–217. DOI: 10.1111/1523-1747.ep12462239

[43] Grattan CE, Boon AP, Eady RA, Winkelmann RK. The pathology of the autologous serum skin test response in chronic urticaria resembles IgE-mediated late-phase reactions. Int Arch Allergy Appl Immunol. 1990;93(2–3): 198–204. DOI: 10.1159/000235301

[44] Kikuchi Y, Kaplan AP. Mechanisms of autoimmune activation of basophils in chronic urticaria. J Allergy Clin Immunol. 2001;107(6):1056–1062. DOI: 10.1067/mai.2001.115484

[45] Konstantinou GN, Asero R, Ferrer M, et al. EAACI taskforce position paper: evidence for autoimmune urticaria and proposal for defining diagnostic criteria. Allergy. 2013;68(1):27–36. DOI: 10.1111/all.12056

[46] Metz M, Ohanyan T, Church MK, Maurer M. Omalizumab is an effective and rapidly acting therapy in difficult-to-treat chronic urticaria: a retrospective

clinical analysis. J Dermatol Sci. 2014;73(1):57–62. DOI: 10.1016/j.jdermsci.2013.08.011

[47] Asero R. Severe CSU and activation of the coagulation/fibrinolysis system: clinical aspects. *Eur Ann Allergy Clin Immunol.* 2019;52(1):15–17. DOI: 10.23822/EurAnnACI.1764-1489.109

[48] Yanase Y, Takahagi S, Hide M. Chronic spontaneous urticaria and the extrinsic coagulation system. Allergol Int. 2018;67(2):191–194. DOI: 10.1016/j.alit.2017.09.003

[49] Saini S, Rosen KE, Hsieh HJ, et al. A randomized, placebo-controlled, dose-ranging study of single-dose omalizumab in patients with H1-antihistamine-refractory chronic idiopathic urticaria. *J Allergy Clin Immunol.* 2011;128(3):567–573.e1. DOI: 10.1016/j.jaci.2011.06.010

[50] Maurer M, Altrichter S, Bieber T, et al. Efficacy and safety of omalizumab in patients with chronic urticaria who exhibit IgE against thyroperoxidase. *J Allergy Clin Immunol.* 2011;128(1):202–209.e5. DOI: 10.1016/j.jaci.2011.04.038

[51] Kaplan AP, Joseph K, Maykut RJ, Geba GP, Zeldin RK. Treatment of chronic autoimmune urticaria with omalizumab. J Allergy Clin Immunol. 2008;122(3):569–573. DOI: 10.1016/j.jaci.2008.07.006

[52] Maurer M, Rosén K, Hsieh HJ, et al. Omalizumab for the treatment of chronic idiopathic or spontaneous urticaria. N Engl J Med. 2013;368:924–935. DOI: 10.1056/NEJMoa1215372

[53] Kaplan A, Ledford D, Ashby M, et al. Omalizumab in patients with symptomatic chronic idiopathic/spontaneous urticaria despite standard combination therapy. J Allergy Clin Immunol. 2013;132(1):101–109. DOI: 10.1016/j.jaci.2013.05.013

[54] Saini SS, Bindslev-Jensen C, Maurer M, et al. Efficacy and safety of omalizumab in patients with chronic idiopathic/spontaneous urticaria who remain symptomatic on H1 antihistamines: a randomized, placebo-controlled study. J Invest Dermatol. 2015;135(1):67–75. DOI: 10.1038/jid.2014.306

[55] Rottem M, Segal R, Kivity S, et al. Omalizumab therapy for chronic spontaneous urticaria: the Israeli experience. Isr Med Assoc J. 2014;16(8):487–490.

[56] Sussman G, Hebert J, Barron C, et al. Real-life experiences with omalizumab for the treatment of chronic urticaria. Ann Allergy Asthma Immunol. 2014;112(2):170–174. DOI: 10.1016/j.anai.2013.12.005

[57] Labrador-Horrillo M, Valero A, Velasco M, et al. Efficacy of omalizumab in chronic spontaneous urticaria refractory to conventional therapy: analysis of 110 patients in real-life practice. Expert Opin Biol Ther. 2013;13(9):1225–1228. DOI: 10.1517/14712598.2013.822484

[58] Giménez-Arnau AM, Toubi E, Marsland AM, Maurer M. Clinical management of urticaria using omalizumab: the first licensed biological therapy available for chronic spontaneous urticaria. J Eur Acad Dermatol Venereol. 2016;30(Suppl 5):25–32. DOI: 10.1111/jdv.13697

[59] Gouveia PM, Gameiro A, Pinho A, Gonçalo M. Long-term management of chronic spontaneous urticaria with omalizumab. Clin Exp Dermatol. 2017;42(7):735–742. DOI: 10.1111/ced.13173

[60] Kaplan A, Ferrer M, Bernstein JA, et al. Timing and duration of omalizumab response in patients with chronic idiopathic/spontaneous urticaria. J Allergy Clin Immunol. 2016;137(2):474–481. DOI: 10.1016/j.jaci.2015.08.023

[61] Vadasz Z, Tal Y, Rotem M, et al. Omalizumab for severe chronic spontaneous urticaria: Real-life experiences of 280 patients. J Allergy Clin Immunol Pract. 2017;5(6):1743–1745. DOI: 10.1016/j.jaip.2017.08.035

[62] Marzano AV, Genovese G, Casazza G, et al. Predictors of response to omalizumab and relapse in chronic spontaneous urticaria: a study of 470 patients. J Eur Acad Dermatol Venereol. 2018;33(5):918–924. DOI: 10.1111/jdv.15350

[63] Giménez-Arnau AM, Santiago AV, Tomás JB, et al. Therapeutic Strategy According to Differences in Response to Omalizumab in Patients With Chronic Spontaneous Urticaria. *J Investig Allergol Clin Immunol.* 2019;29(5):338–348. DOI: 10.18176/jiaci.0323

[64] Eghrari-Sabet J, Sher E, Kavati A, et al. Real-world use of omalizumab in patients with chronic idiopathic/spontaneous urticaria in the United State. Allergy Asthma Proc. 2018;39(3): 191–200. DOI: 10.2500/aap.2018.39.4132

[65] Hide M, Park HS, Igarashi A, et al. Efficacy and safety of omalizumab in Japanese and Korean patients with refractory chronic spontaneous urticaria. J Dermatol Sci. 2017;87(1):70–78. DOI: 10.1016/j.jdermsci.2017.03.009

[66] Zhao ZT, Ji CM, Yu WJ, et al. Omalizumab for the treatment of chronic spontaneous urticaria: A meta-analysis of randomized clinical trials. *J Allergy Clin Immunol.* 2016;137(6): 1742–1750.e4. DOI: 10.1016/j.jaci.2015.12.1342

[67] Ensina LF, Valle SO, Juliani AP, et al. Omalizumab in chronic spontaneous urticaria: a Brazilian real-life experience. Int Arch Allergy Immunol. 2016;169(2):121–124. DOI: 10.1159/000444985

[68] Ghazanfar MN, Sand C, Thomsen SF. Effectiveness and safety of omalizumab in chronic spontaneous or inducible urticaria: evaluation of 154 patients. Br J Dermatol. 2016;175(2): 404–406. DOI: 10.1111/bjd.14540

[69] Giménez-Arnau A, Velasco M, Armario Hita JC, Labrador-Horrillo M, Silvestre Salvador JF. Omalizumab: what benefits should we expect? Eur J Dermatol. 2016;26(4):340–344. DOI: 10.1684/ejd.2016.2809.

[70] Metz M, Ohanyan T, Church MK, Maurer M. Retreatment with omalizumab results in rapid remission in chronic spontaneous and inducible urticaria. JAMA Dermatol. 2014;150(3): 288–290. DOI: 10.1001/jamadermatol.2013.8705

[71] Metz M, Staubach P, Bauer A, et al. Clinical efficacy of omalizumab in chronic spontaneous urticaria is associated with a reduction of FcεRI-positive cells in the skin. Theranostics. 2017;7(5):1266–1276. DOI: 10.7150/thno.18304

[72] Savic S, Marsland A, McKay D, et al. Retrospective case note review of chronic spontaneous urticaria outcomes and adverse effects in patients treated with omalizumab or ciclosporin in UK secondary care. Allergy Asthma Clin Immunol. 2015;11(1):21. DOI: 10.1186/s13223-015-0088-7.

[73] Song CH, Stern S, Giruparajah M, Berlin N, Sussman GL. Long-term efficacy of fixed-dose omalizumab for patients with severe chronic spontaneous urticaria. Ann Allergy Asthma Immunol. 2013;110(2):113–117. DOI: 10.1016/j.anai.2012.11.022

[74] Türk M, Yilmaz I, Bahcecioglu SN. Treatment and retreatment with omalizumab in chronic spontaneous urticaria: real life experience with twenty-five patients. Allergol Int. 2017; 67(1):85–89. DOI: 10.1016/j.alit.2017.05.003

[75] Grzanka R, Damasiewicz-Bodzek A, Kasperska-Zajac A. Interplay between acute phase response and coagulation/ fibrinolysis in chronic spontaneous urticaria. Allergy Asthma Clin Immunol. 2018;14:27. DOI: 10.1186/s13223-018-0255-8

[76] Weller K, Ohanyan T, Hawro T, et al. Total IgE levels are linked to the response of chronic spontaneous urticaria patients to omalizumab. Allergy. 2018;73(12):2406–2408. DOI: 10.1111/all.13586

[77] Gericke J, Metz M, Ohanyan T, et al. Serum autoreactivity predicts time to response to omalizumab therapy in chronic spontaneous urticaria. *J Allergy Clin Immunol.* 2017;139(3):1059–1061.e1. DOI: 10.1016/j.jaci.2016.07.047

[78] Palacios T, Stillman L, Borish L, Lawrence M. Lack of basophil CD203c-upregulating activity as an immunological marker to predict response to treatment with omalizumab in patients with symptomatic chronic urticaria. J Allergy Clinical Immunol Pract. 2016;4(3):529–530. DOI: 10.1016/j.jaip.2015.11.025

[79] Clayton E, Saltoun CA. Clinical Predictors of Response to Omalizumab for Treatment of Chronic Urticaria. J Allergy Clin Immunol. 2017;139(2):AB244. DOI: 10.1016/j.jaci.2016.12.785

[80] Ghazanfar MN, Sand C, Thomsen SF. Effectiveness and safety of omalizumab in chronic spontaneous or inducible urticaria: evaluation of 154 patients. Br J Dermatol. 2016;175(2):404–406. DOI: 10.1111/bjd.14540

[81] Asero R Canonica GW, Cristaudo A, et al. Critical appraisal of the unmet needs in the treatment of chronic spontaneous urticaria with omalizumab: an Italian perspective. Curr Opin Allergy Clin Immunol. 2017;17(6):453–459. DOI: 10.1097/ACI.0000000000000404

[82] Ferrer M, Boccon-Gibod I, Gonçalo M, et al. Expert opinion: defining response to omalizumab in patients with chronic spontaneous urticaria. Eur J Dermatol. 2017;27(5):455–463. DOI: 10.1684/ejd.2017.3085

[83] Tharp MD, Bernstein JA, Kavati A, et al. Benefits and Harms of Omalizumab Treatment in Adolescent and Adult Patients With Chronic Idiopathic (Spontaneous) Urticaria: A Meta-analysis of "Real-world" Evidence. JAMA Dermatol. 2019;155(1):29–38. DOI: 10.1001/jamadermatol.2018.3447

[84] Maurer M, Weller K, Bindslev-Jensen C, et al. Unmet clinical needs in chronic spontaneous urticaria. A GA^{2}LEN task force report. Allergy. 2011;66(3):317–330. DOI: 10.1111/j.1398-9995.2010.02496.x

[85] Sussman G, Hébert J, Gulliver W, et al. Omalizumab Re-Treatment and Step-Up in Patients with Chronic Spontaneous Urticaria: OPTIMA Trial. *J Allergy Clin Immunol Pract.* 2020;8(7):2372–2378.e5. DOI: 10.1016/j.jaip.2020.03.022.

[86] Maurer M, Kaplan A, Rosén K, et al. The XTEND-CIU study: Long-term use of omalizumab in chronic idiopathic urticaria. *J Allergy Clin Immunol.* 2018; 141(3):1138–1139.e7. DOI: 10.1016/j.jaci.2017.10.018

[87] Chen Y, Yu M, Huang X. Omalizumab treatment and outcomes in Chinese patients with chronic spontaneous urticaria, chronic inducible urticaria, or both. World Allergy Organ J. 2021;14(1):100501. DOI: 10.1016/j.waojou.2020.100501

[88] Arm JP, Bottoli I, Skerjanec A, et al. Pharmacokinetics, pharmacodynamics and safety of QGE031 (ligelizumab), a novel high-affinity anti-IgE antibody, in atopic subjects. Clin Exp Allergy. 2014; 44(11):1371–1385. DOI: 10.1111/cea.12400

[89] Busse W, Corren J, Lanier BQ, et al. Omalizumab, anti-IgE recombinant humanized monoclonal antibody, for the treatment of severe allergic asthma. J Allergy Clin Immunol. 2001;108(2): 184–190. DOI: 10.1067/mai.2001.117880

[90] Gauvreau GM, Arm JP, Boulet L-P, et al. Efficacy and safety of multiple doses of QGE031 (ligelizumab) versus omalizumab and placebo in inhibiting allergen-induced early asthmatic responses. J Allergy Clin Immunol. 2016;138(4):1051–1059. DOI: 10.1016/j.jaci.2016.02.027

[91] Gasser P, Tarchevskaya SS, Guntern P, et al. The mechanistic and functional profile of the therapeutic anti-IgE antibody ligelizumab differs from omalizumab. Nat Commun. 2020; 11(1):165. DOI: 10.1038/s41467-019-13815-w

[92] Gould HJ, Sutton BJ. IgE in allergy and asthma today. Nat Rev Immunol. 2008;8(3), 205–217. DOI: 10.1038/nri2273

[93] Coyle AJ, Wagner K, Bertrand C, Tsuyuki S, Bews J, Heusser C. Central role of immunoglobulin (Ig) E in the induction of lung eosinophil infiltration and T helper 2 cell cytokine production: inhibition by a non-anaphylactogenic anti-IgE antibody. J Exp Med. 1996;183 (4):1303–1310. DOI: 10.1084/jem.183.4.1303

[94] Maurer M, Giménez-Arnau AM, Sussman G, et al. Ligelizumab for chronic spontaneous urticaria. N Engl J Med. 2019;381 (14):1321–1332. DOI: 10.1056/NEJMoa190040898

[95] Bernstein JA, Baker D, Maurer M, et al. Ligelizumab achieves sustained control of chronic spontaneous urticaria symptoms of hives, itch and angioedema: 1-year treatment results. Allergy. 2019;74(S106):21. DOI: 10.1111/all.1395799.

[96] Soong W, Metz M, Bernstein JA, et al. Long-term treatment with ligelizumab achieves prolonged symptom control in patients with chronic spontaneous urticaria during the post-treatment follow-up. J Allergy Clin Immunol. 2020;145(2):AB341. DOI: 10.1016/j.jaci.2019.12.077100

[97] Giménez-Arnau AM, Salman A. Targeted Therapy for Chronıc Spontaneous Urtıcarıa: Ratıonale and Recent Progress. Drugs. 2020;80(16): 1617–1634. DOI: 10.1007/s40265-020-01387-9

[98] Severin T, Maurer M, Giménez-Arnau AM, et al. Study design and rationale of a phase 3b extension study of ligelizumab in adult and adolescent patients with chronic spontaneous urticaria. Allergy. 2020;75(S109):446. DOI: 10.1111/all.14508

[99] Ensina LF, Cusato-Ensina AP, Camelo-Nunes IC, Solé D. Omalizumab as third-line therapy for urticaria during pregnancy. *J Investig Allergol Clin Immunol*. 2017;27(5):326–327. DOI: 10.18176/jiaci.0179

[100] Ghazanfar MN, Thomsen SF. Successful and safe treatment of chronic spontaneous urticaria with omalizumab in a woman during two consecutive pregnancies. Case Rep Med. 2015;2015: 368053. DOI:10.1155/2015/36805350.

[101] Gonzalez-Medina M, Curto-Barredo L, Labrador-Horrillo M, Giménez-Arnau A. Omalizumab use during pregnancy for chronic spontaneous urticaria (CSU): report of two cases. J Eur Acad Dermatol Venereol. 2017;31(5):e245-e246. DOI: 10.1111/jdv.14034

[102] Namazy JA, Blais L, Andrews EB, et al. Pregnancy outcomes in the omalizumab pregnancy registry and a disease-matched comparator cohort. *J Allergy Clin Immunol.* 2020;145(2):528–536.e1. DOI: 10.1016/j.jaci.2019.05.019

[103] Passanisi S, Arasi S, Caminiti L, Crisafulli G, Salzano G, Pajno GB. Omalizumab in children and adolescents with chronic spontaneous urticaria: case series and review of the literature. Dermatol Ther. 2020;33(4): e13489. DOI: 10.1111/dth.13489

[104] Ari A, Levy Y, Segal N, et al. Efficacy of omalizumab treatment for pediatric chronic spontaneous urticaria: a multi-center retrospective case series. Pediatr Dermatol. 2020;37(6):1051–1054. DOI: 10.1111/pde.1436042

[105] Nettis E, Cegolon L, Di Leo E, Canonica WG, Detoraki A, Italian OCUReL Study Group. Omalizumab in elderly patients with chronic spontaneous urticaria: An Italian real-life experience. Ann Allergy Asthma Immunol. 2018;120(3):318–323. DOI: 10.1016/j.anai.2017.12.007

[106] Vollono L, Piccolo A, Lanna C, et al. Omalizumab for chronic spontaneous urticaria in "complex" patients: data from real-life clinical practice. Drug Des Devel Ther. 2019;13: 3181–3186. DOI:10.2147/DDDT. S21430766

[107] Larenas-Linnemann D, Saini SS, Azamar-Jácome AA, Maurer M. Chronic urticaria can be caused by cancer and resolves with its cure. Allergy. 2018;73 (7):1562–1566. DOI:10.1111/all.13434

[108] Türk M, Carneiro-Leão L, Kolkhir P, Bonnekoh H, Buttgereit T, Maurer M. How to treat patients with chronic spontaneous urticaria with omalizumab: questions and answers. J Allergy Clin Immunol Pract. 2020;8(1): 113–124. DOI: 10.1016/j.jaip.2019.07.021

[109] Kocatürk E, Zuberbier T. New biologics in the treatment of urticaria. Curr Opin Allergy Clin Immunol. 2018; 18(5):425–431. DOI: 10.1097/ ACI.0000000000000466

[110] Scheerens H, Putnam W, Zheng Y, et al. Treatment with MEMP1972A, an anti-M1 prime monoclonal antibody, reduced serum IgE in healthy volunteers and patients with allergic rhinitis. Am J Respir Crit Care Med. 2012;185: A6791.109.

[111] Gauvreau GM, Harris JM, Boulet LP, et al. Targeting membrane-expressed IgE B cell receptor with an antibody to the M1 prime epitope reduces IgE production. *Sci Transl Med.* 2014;6(243):243ra85. DOI: 10.1126/ scitranslmed.3008961

[112] Harris JM, Cabanski CR, Scheerens H, et al. A randomized trial of quilizumab in adults with refractory chronic spontaneous urticaria. J Allergy Clin Immunol. 2016;138(6):1730–1732. DOI: 10.1016/j.jaci.2016.06.023111

[113] Ferrer M, Nakazawa K, Kaplan AP. Complement dependence of histamine release in chronic urticaria. J Allergy Clin Immunol. 1999;104(1):169-172. DOI: 10.1016/s0091-6749(99)70129-6

[114] Kikuchi Y, Kaplan AP. A role for C5a in augmenting IgG-dependent histamine release from basophils in chronic urticaria. J Allergy Clin Immunol. 2002;109(1):114–118. DOI: 10.1067/mai.2002.120954

[115] Korosec P, Subic T, Adamic K, Silar M, Kosnik M. C5a-induced in vitro basophil activation in patients with chronic urticaria: a pilot study. Wien Klin Wochenschr. 2009;121(9–10):339–343. DOI: 10.1007/s00508-009-1168-9

[116] Huber M, Helgason CD, Damen JE, Liu L, Humphries RK, Krystal G. The src homology 2-containing inositol phosphatase (SHIP) is the gatekeeper of mast cell degranulation. Proc Natl Acad Sci USA. 1998;95(19):11330–11335. DOI: 10.1073/pnas.95.19.1133

[117] Cherwinski HM, Murphy CA, Joyce BL, et al. The CD200 receptor is a novel and potent regulator of murine and human mast cell function. J

Immunol. 2005;174:1348–1356. DOI: 10.4049/jimmunol.174.3.1348

[118] Zampeli E, Tiligada E. The role of histamine H4 receptor in immune and inflammatory disorders. Br J Pharmacol. 2009;157:24–33. DOI: 10.1111/ j.1476-5381.2009.00151.x

[119] Cowden JM, Zhang M, Dunford PJ, Thurmond RL. The histamine H4 receptor mediates inflammation and pruritus in Th2-dependent dermal inflammation. J Invest Dermatol. 2010; 130(4):1023–1033. DOI: 10.1038/ jid.2009.358

[120] Werfel T, Layton G, Yeadon M, et al. Efficacy and safety of the histamine H4 receptor antagonist ZPL-3893787 in patients with atopic dermatitis. *J Allergy Clin Immunol.* 2019; 143(5):1830–1837.e4. DOI: 10.1016/j. jaci.2018.07.047

[121] Gangemi S, Quartuccio S, Casciaro M, Trapani G, Minciullo PL, Imbalzano E. Interleukin 31 and skin diseases: a systematic review. Allergy Asthma Proc. 2017;38:401–408. DOI: 10.2500/aap.2017.38.4080

[122] Luo XY, Liu Q, Yang H, et al. OSMR gene effect on the pathogenesis of chronic autoimmune Urticaria via the JAK/STAT3 pathway. Mol Med. 2018;24 (1):28. DOI: 10.1186/s10020-018-0025-6

[123] Kasperska-Zajac A, Sztylc J, Machura E, Jop G. Plasma IL-6 concentration correlates with clinical disease activity and serum C-reactive protein concentration in chronic urticaria patients. Clin Exp Allergy. 2011;41(10):1386–1391. DOI: 10.1111/ j.1365-2222.2011.03789.x.

[124] Krause K, Feist E, Fiene M, Kallinich T, Maurer M. Complete remission in 3 of 3 anti-IL-6-treated patients with Schnitzler syndrome. J Allergy Clin Immunol. 2012;129(3):848–850. DOI: 10.1016/j.jaci.2011.10.031

[125] Fujisawa D, Kashiwakura J-I, Kita H, et al. Expression of Mas-related gene X2 on mast cells is upregulated in the skin of patients with severe chronic urticaria. *J Allergy Clin Immunol.* 2014; 134(3):622–633.e9. DOI: 10.1016/j. jaci.2014.05.004

[126] Ständer S, Siepmann D, Herrgott I, Sunderkötter C, Luger TA. Targeting the neurokinin receptor 1 with aprepitant: a novel antipruritic strategy. PLoS One. 2010;5(6):e10968. DOI: 10.1371/journal.pone.0010968

[127] Takai T. TSLP expression: cellular sources, triggers, and regulatory mechanisms. Allergol Int. 2012;61:3–17. DOI: 10.2332/allergolint.11-RAI-0395

[128] Yan S, Chen W, Zhang Y, Li J, Chen X. Calcium release-activated calcium modulator 1 as a therapeutic target in allergic skin diseases. Life Sci. 2019;228:152–157. DOI: 10.1016/j. lfs.2019.05.001

[129] Li J, Guo A, Chen W, et al. Association of ORAI1 gene polymorphisms with chronic spontaneous urticaria and the efficacy of the nonsedating H1 antihistamine desloratadine. *J Allergy Clin Immunol.* 2017;139(4):1386–1388.e9. DOI: 10.1016/j.jaci.2016.10.017

[130] Metz M, Torene R, Kaiser S, et al. Omalizumab normalizes the gene expression signature of lesional skin in patients with chronic spontaneous urticaria: a randomized, double-blind, placebo-controlled study. Allergy. 2019; 74(1):141–151. DOI: 10.1111/all.13547118

[131] Staubach P, Metz M, Chapman-Rothe N, et al. Effect of omalizumab on angioedema in H1 -antihistamine-resistant chronic spontaneous urticaria patients: results from X-ACT, a randomized controlled trial. Allergy.

2016;71(8):1135–1144. DOI: 10.1111/all.12870119

[132] Staubach P, Metz M, Chapman-Rothe N, et al. Omalizumab rapidly improves angioedema-related quality of life in adult patients with chronic spontaneous urticaria: X-ACT study data. Allergy. 2018;73(3):576–584. DOI: 10.1111/all.13339

[133] Hide M, Igarashi A, Yagami A, et al. Efficacy and safety of omalizumab for the treatment of refractory chronic spontaneous urticaria in japanese patients: subgroup analysis of the phase 3 POLARIS study. Allergol Int. 2018;67(2):243–252. DOI: 10.1016/j.alit.2017.10.001

[134] Maurer M, Schutz A, Weller K, et al. Omalizumab is effective in symptomatic dermographism-results of a randomized placebo-controlled trial. *J Allergy Clin Immunol.* 2017;140(3):870–873.e5. DOI: 10.1016/j.jaci.2017.01.042

[135] Gastaminza G, Azofra J, Nunez-Cordoba JM, et al. Efficacy and safety of omalizumab (xolair) for cholinergic urticaria in patients unresponsive to a double dose of antihistamines: a randomized mixed double-blind and open-label placebo-controlled clinical trial. *J Allergy Clin Immunol Pract.* 2019;7(5):1599–1609.e1. DOI: 10.1016/j.jaip.2018.12.025

[136] Metz M, Schutz A, Weller K, et al. Omalizumab is effective in cold urticaria-results of a randomized placebo-controlled trial. *J Allergy Clin Immunol.* 2017;140(3):864–867.e5. DOI: 10.1016/j.jaci.2017.01.043

[137] Aubin F, Avenel-Audran M, Jeanmougin M, et al. Omalizumab in patients with severe and refractory solar urticaria: a Phase II multicentric study. J Am Acad Dermatol. 2016;74(3):574–575. DOI: 10.1016/j.jaad.2015.11.021124

Chapter 6

New Biological Treatment Options in CSU

Zahava Vadasz and Elias Toubi

Abstract

Chronic spontaneous urticaria (CSU) is a devastating disease and is associated with many co-morbidities and long-lasting suffering. Therefore, patients always look for a most efficient therapeutic approach to achieve a full remission. In many patients, CSU remain refractory to off-label doses of antihistamines and short courses of steroids, and therefore are treated with omalizumab. However, 15–20% of severe CSU patients will stay unresponsive to omalizumab and are defined as being of un-met needs. In this review we will shed light on the many new drugs which are assessed in ongoing clinical trials.

Keywords: Chronic spontaneous urticaria, T-cells, autoimmunity, treatment

1. Introduction

Chronic spontaneous urticarial (CSU) with or without angioedema, is a condition which lasts more than 6 weeks, without an apparent trigger. It results from a pathogenic over-activation of dermal mast cells and basophils, followed by their degranulation and the release of pro-inflammatory mediators (mainly histamine) inducing the appearance of transient itchy wheals, and occasionally episodes of angioedema. The prevalence of CSU is estimated to be between 0.5-1percent in the general population, with an incidence of 0.10 to 1.50 per 1000 person-years. It predominantly affects female, with symptom onset occurring mainly between 20 and 40 years [1]. Earlier studies reported on CSU lasting over one year in more than 70% of cases and continuing to exist in 14% of them after five years. CSU duration was associated with the presence of angioedema and disease severity. In a recent study, younger CSU patients (22 ± 16 years) tended to have a significantly longer course, were in 16% of patients, CSU symptoms lasted over ten years [2, 3]. In addition to its prolonged duration, CSU severely affects quality of life and is associated with comorbidities such as lack of sleep, impairments in work productivity, and depression/anxiety. In one study about 50% of patients with CSU were diagnosed with one or more psychosomatic disorders, the most frequent of which was anxiety, followed by depressive and somatoform disorders [4, 5]. The prevalence of rheumatoid arthritis, systemic lupus erythematosus, thyroiditis and vitiligo were found to be significantly increased in CSU patients [6]. Patients without any evidence of comorbidities at the time of their CSU diagnosis had an increased risk of developing mast cell-mediated diseases including atopic diseases [7]. Many studies have focused on the importance of clinical and laboratory biomarkers for the assessment of CSU severity and the evaluation of treatment efficacy. Clinical manifestations such as asthma and thyroid disease were associated with higher disease severity and duration [8]. Laboratory markers, namely, C-reactive protein (CRP), autologous serum skin test (ASST), basophil activation test (BAT, D-dimer levels and total serum IgE are all potential blood biomarkers that are useful for CSU management [9]. Many CSU patients continue to suffer from symptoms of pruritus, urticaria, and angioedema despite the acceptable up dosing of second-generation antihistamines (up to fourfold) [10]. Recurrent short courses of steroids were also reported to have only a short-term beneficial effect in severe CSU patients. Current treatments are considerably effective in achieving good response and favorable remission, however, many CSU patients are still refractory to these available treatments. This is why, it is extremely important to identify and understand underlying disease mechanisms, in order to achieve better therapeutic outcomes. In addition to a brief summary covering the pathogenesis of CSU, and the currently used therapies, this chapter will focus on emerging new therapies, some of which are being studied in on-going clinical trials, and others that are being assessed as potential candidates for treatment.

2. Pathophysiology

At the very beginning (four decades ago), CSU was considered to be a T-cell mediated disorder, supported by the finding of rich CD4+ T-cell infiltration in the skin of CSU patients [11]. The involvement of activated T-cells in peripheral blood of CSU patients, namely the increased expression of CD40 ligand on T-cells similarly to what we find on activated T-cells from patients suffering from active systemic lupus erythematosus and other autoimmune diseases was also reported [12]. In concert with this, there are studies showing an increased switch of Th1 to Th17 in the peripheral blood of CSU patients in correlation with CSU disease severity, and IL-17 levels are significantly higher in the autologous serum skin test (ASST) positive than ASST negative CSU patients. Plasma levels of interferon-γ (IFN-γ), IL-2 and IL-21 were also found to be significantly higher in ASST-positive CSU subgroups, known to involve the positive regulation of the Janus-kinase-signal transducer and activator of transcription (JAK/STAT) signaling pathway [13]. In a recent study using Kunming mice (a model of CSU), a longer duration and higher intensity of pruritus was demonstrated to be in association with enhanced levels of eosinophils, inflammatory cytokine expression and activated the JAK/STAT signaling pathway. This was found to be in mice overexpressing IL-9 and IL-10, contributing to the development of CSU by signaling the JAK/STAT pathway [14]. Commensurate with this, is the later finding of antigen/disease-specific auto-reactive CD4 + T cells that target FcεRIα in most patients with CSU, with a cytokine secretion profile typical of aTh1 immune response. This is compatible with the earlier finding of IgG autoantibodies to FcεRIα on dermal mast cells and basophils, supporting the concept that CSU is an autoimmune disorder probably mediated by auto-reactive T cells. IFN-γ and autoantibody responses to FcεRIα were found to be inversely related, with IFN-γ responses being detected earlier than autoantibodies in the course of CSU. This finding of inverse relationship between auto-reactive T-cell responses and autoimmunity suggests these responses to be different stages in the pathogenesis of CSU [15]. In a very recent study we found that increased numbers of CD4 + T cells and mast cells were present in both lesional and non-lesional skin of CSU patients when compared with the healthy controls. Both types of cells were strongly positive for IL-17A and found to be in close proximity to each other [16]. With respect to the aforementioned, autoimmunity in CSU patients is reported to be found in at least 50% of cases. Two types of autoimmunity have been documented and supported by numerous reports. The first (type I) is driven by

IgE auto-antibodies against thyroid antigens and/or auto-allergens, defined by the presence of anti-TPO antibodies. In parallel to this, is the finding of type IIb auto-immunity characterized by the binding of IgG auto-antibodies (recently also IgA and Ig M) to IgE and/or FcεRIα on mast cells [17–19]. Both types are followed by the intense activation and degranulation of mast cells and the release of inflammatory mediators in the skin that are able to induce itchy wheals and angioedema. Among the many mediated agents, histamine, pro-inflammatory cytokines and chemokines are the most frequent [20]. Basophils and Eosinophils have recently been included among other cells actively involved in the pathogenesis of CSU. In this respect, peripheral blood basopenia is frequently reported in association with CSU disease severity. It has been postulated that this is a result of the migration of basophils from blood to the skin of active CSU patients. Basopenia resolves in parallel with CSU remission and therefore may become a suitable marker for follow-up [21]. Recent evidence suggests that eosinophils may also play role in the pathogenesis of CSU. Both eosinophils and eosinophil granules were displayed in lesional skin of CSU patients. This is in contrast to allergic rhinitis and asthma where peripheral blood eosinophilia is a characteristic finding, while in CSU, peripheral blood eosinopenia is observed in association with disease severity. As in the case of basopenia, depletion of active eosinophils and their shift to the skin of CSU patients is the most accepted mechanism of this phenomenon [22]. The issue of how all these cells, and mechanisms, are linked, and how they act at onset or during the persistence of CSU is extremely complex. However, current therapies, targeting free IgE, mast cells and T cells are reported to be tremendously efficient in inducing CSU remission.

3. Current therapies for CSU

The introduction of the non-sedative anti-histamines replacing the first generation (sedative) one was a giant step forward in the treatment of CSU. At a later date, H1-antihistamine up-dosing was established and shown to be safe and of better efficacy. However, even when up-dosing was increased fourfold, the rate of non-responders remained high, thereby suggesting that additional treatments were needed [23]. As early as 1991, targeting T-cells by cyclosporine A (CsA) was shown to be highly effective in severe cases of CSU [24]. Later on, we demonstrated that low doses of CsA (2–3 mg/ml) given for three months were both extremely beneficial and had a low prevalence of side-effects. In some patients, we could demonstrate a long-lasting full remission, while in others it was even curative [25]. The efficacy of CsA was established by many double-blind, randomized studies. Symptom scores significantly improved in the CsA group over with placebo. CsA was well tolerated at daily doses of 3 mg/kg. Side effects such as hypertension and increased serum creatinine were rare [26]. In addition, the efficacy and safety of CsA in CSU was evaluated by a meta-analysis of eighteen studies. A low-dose (2–3 mg/kg/d) was considered to be both beneficial and safe, and adverse events appear to be dose dependent and occur more frequently in patients that have been treated with moderate doses (4–5 mg/kg/d) [27]. In a recent study, the prediction of beneficial response to CsA treatment, was assessed using, positive ASST, plasma D-dimer levels, IL-2, IL-5 levels and total IgE level. Decreased plasma D-dimer levels, and decreased serum IL-2 and IL-5were reported to be correlated with clinical improvement after CsA treatment [28]. While cyclosporine A is still used in cases with severe CSU, the fear of side effects, mainly in those with mild hypertension or diabetes, has limited its usage, allowing omalizumab (an IgG-anti-IgE monoclonal antibody), approved for the treatment of anti-histamine-refractory CSU in 2014 to become the preferable option in treating CSU. In the European

Academy of Allergology and Clinical Immunology, Global Allergy and Asthma European Network, European Dermatology Forum, and World Allergy (EAACI/GA2LEN/EDF/WAO) guidelines for the treatment of CSU, it is recommended that omalizumab should be added to off-label doses of anti-histamines when CSU is inadequately controlled [29, 30]. Cyclosporine A remains the final option for those considered to be omalizumab failures. The main mechanism through which omalizumab acts, is its ability to bind soluble IgE and the down regulation of FcεRI expression on skin mast cells. This is followed by decreased mast cell activation and degranulation. In this respect, higher levels of FcεRI expression, predict a faster response to omalizumab. In addition higher levels of total serum IgE were shown to be associated with a greater responsiveness to omalizumab [31]. While it is well accepted that a complete response to the standard dose of omalizumab (300 mg/month) is observed in about 59% of patients, 15% of treated patients still remain resistant to this dose of omalizumab [32]. In many studies, up dosing of omalizumab to 450 mg/month was shown to achieve better clinical respnses with a good safety profile [33]. Options of higher doses of cyclosporine A or the combination of omalizumab and cyclosporine A were also reported in few case reports in severe and refractory to all of the above mentioned approaches. Un-met needs and the requirement for new treatments in still refractory CSU are the subject of many on-going clinical trials in which targeting new relevant pathways is assessed.

4. New drugs in ongoing clinical trials

4.1 Anti IgE

4.1.1 Ligelizumab

Ligelizumab (QGE031) is a new monoclonal antibody directed against the Cε3 domain of IgE, which in preclinical and in phase I clinical studies demonstrated its 50-fold greater affinity to IgE in vitro and six- to nine-fold greater potency in vivo compared to omalizumab. This affinity difference is caused due to epitope differences between ligelizumab and omalizumab that contribute to their distinct qualitative IgE-receptor profiles. Ligelizumab was superior in its ability to suppress IgE binding to FcεRI, basophil activation, and IgE secretion by B cells [34]. It was also shown that Ligelizumab provided a longer suppression of free and cell-bound IgE [35]. Omalizumab was shown to inhibit the interaction of IgE-FcεRII (CD23) more efficiently than Omalizumb, and this finding might explain the superior anti-asthmatic effect of omalizumb, considering the role of CD23 in lung inflammation [34]. In order to further assess its efficacy in CSU, a phase IIb dose-finding trial was designed for the efficacy and safety of ligelizumab. Doses of 24 mg, 72 mg, and 240 mg every four weeks were compared to the omalizumab standard dose of 300 mg every four weeks and to placebo in 382 adult patients with CSU. Clinical beneficial effects were evaluated by using - UAS7 (Urticaria Activity Score) and HSS7 (Hives Severity Score). The percentage of patients with a complete control of their hives (HSS7:0) and a complete control of their symptoms (UAS7:0) at week 12 was significantly higher in all ligelizumab arms (24 mg, 72 mg, 240 mg) compared with omalizumab (300 mg) and the placebo. The question regarding the low complete response rates with omalizumab was attributed to the high percentage of patients with an autoimmune pattern and angioedema. Adverse events rates were similar in all groups, except for a slightly higher incidence of local reaction at the injection site of ligelizumab 240 mg compared to omalizumab [36]. Patient's follow up in this clinical study revealed that among patients who achieved an UAS7 ≤ 6 at week 20, the beneficial therapeutic response was maintained for a median of 16, 8 and 8 weeks with ligelizumab 240 mg, 72 mg, and omalizumab, respectively. In addition, a 1-year extension phase of the above clinical study showed that in patients with UAS7 ≥ 12 who received ligelizumab 240 mg every 4 weeks (NCT02649218), the UAS7 ≤ 6 score response was maintained for a median period of 28 weeks [37]. Moreover, the treatment with ligelizumab was superior in other clinical measures when compared with omalizumab, namely, a decrease in the use of rescue medication [38] a greater and sustained efficacy in reducing angioedema at week 12 (the percentage of angioedema-free patients with ligelizumab 72 mg, 240 mg, omalizumab 300 mg, and placebo, was 87.5%, 94.9%, 76.3%, and 68.3%, respectively [39]. Several Phase III clinical trials (NCT03580356, NCT03580369, NCT03437278, NCT04210843) are currently in progress in order to further investigate the efficacy and safety of ligelizumab 72 mg and 120 mg when compared with omalizumab 300 mg and a placebo in CSU adolescent and adult patients up to 52 weeks. In Japan, in adult CSU patients who failed to response to H1-anti-histamines, are part of another phase III, open-label, and single-arm study of ligelizumab that is currently in progress (NCT03907878). It is hopeful that these studies and the extension phase study with ligelizumab will better characterize its usage in re-treatment, and self-administration, as well as its its benefit as a monotherapy.

4.1.2 UB-221

Another new monoclonal antibody against IgE, UB-221, has up to eightfold greater affinity for free IgE in comparison with omalizumab. This new compound is currently being investigated for safety, tolerability, pharmacodynamics and pharmacokinetics in an ongoing phase I clinical trial in adult patients with CSU. The study is composed of single doses [0.2, 0.6, 2, 6, 10 mg/kg UB-221] given intravenously (IV) vs. a placebo (NCT03632291, NCT04175704) [40].

4.2 B cells

4.2.1 Bruton's tyrosine kinase (BTK) inhibitors

Bruton tyrosine kinase (BTK) is a tyrosine kinase which was found to play a major role in B cell development. At a later date, it was found to be expressed in various hematopoietic cells including macrophages, mast cells, and basophils. In the context of CSU pathogenesis, BTK was also found to play a major role in the FcεR activation and signaling in mast cells [41, 42]. BTK inhibitors are widely used today to treat several B cell malignancies and auto immune disorders [43]. Out of the many known BTK inhibitors, four (ibrutinib, dasatinib, AVL-292, CNX-774) are recognized to be effective suppressors of IgE-induced activation and histamine release from basophils and mast cells [44]. Ibrutinib (420 mg/day), was assessed in patients suffering from peanut/tree nut allergy and reported to suppress skin test responses to these food allergens within seven days, and without any discernable adverse events. No serious adverse events 100. Upon considering of the pivotal role of FcεRI signaling in CSU, it seems that the use of BTK inhibitors for CSU could be a potential new treatment option. LOU064 (remibrutinib), a more selective BTK inhibitor is being investigated in ongoing phase II clinical trials (NCT03926611, NCT04109313) for its efficacy and safety in adult patients with CSU. In an in-vitro study, the binding of BTK by remibrunitib was more efficient than fenebrutinib, thus it has a faster onset of action and its effects are maintained longer [45]. Another phase II study, investigating a new BTK inhibitor (fenebrutinib 200 mg orally twice a day), in adult patients suffering from CSU, has recently been completed. The results of this study indicated that at week 8, a marked improvement of the UAS7 was achieved at 200 mg twice a day compared with the placebo group [33].

4.2.2 Anti-CD20

Rituximab (RTX) is a well-known monoclonal antibody directed against CD20. It causes the depletion of mature and memory B cells through several mechanisms such as CDC and ADCC. For many years, it has been used to treat B cell hematological malignancies and autoimmune diseases such as- rheumatoid arthritis (RA), and pemphigus vulgaris [46]. Due to the autoimmune nature of CSU, it seems reasonable that the reduction of memory B cells and a subsequent decrease of the autoantibodies due to Rituximab, could well become a beneficial treatment option, particularly in autoimmune CSU. So far, only five patients in whom severe CSU refractory to immunosuppressive treatments, have been treated with rituximab [47–51]. The treatment regimen in these patients was either as used in lymphoma (375 mg/m2 weekly for 4 weeks) or as used in the RA protocol (two doses of 1000 mg with a 2-week interval). Four patients responded well to this treatment, and only one failed. However, a phase I/II open-label trial (NCT00216762) was terminated due to safety concerns. To date, there are no ongoing clinical trials on Rituximab in CSU patients. It appears that Rituximab could be reserved for future use as an alternative treatment option in patients with very severe, and treatment-resistant CSU.

4.3 Basophils, eosinophils and Th2 cells

4.3.1 Chemo attractant receptor-homologous molecule expressed on Th2 (CRTH2) inhibitors

CRTH2 is the prostaglandin D2 (PGD2) receptor that is secreted from mast cells upon activation and degranulation. CRTH2 is normally expressed on eosinophils, basophils, and Th2 cells. The signaling pathways following PGD2-interaction\ligation to CRTH2 results in the stimulation and chemotaxis of basophils and eosinophils, Th2 response, and the increase in the amount of histamine released from basophils [52, 53]. In patients suffering from CSU, membrane CRTH2 expression on basophils and eosinophils, was found to be extremely low, which was presumably attributed to the internalization of CRTH2 upon PGD2 binding. These results suggested a role for PGD2 via CRTH2 ligation in CSU [54]. A particular CRTH2 gene polymorphism was demonstrated in several patients suffering from CSU, and these specific patients needed high doses of anti-histamines in order to control CSU [53]. These findings further establish a role for CRTH2 in CSU pathogenesis, suggesting the relevance of its targeting. Based on these considerations, a new oral CRTH2 antagonist, AZD1981, was generated and used for the treatment of CSU in a clinical trial. In a phase II, double-blind, placebo-controlled trial, twenty-six CSU patients were enrolled and completed the 4-week treatment period with either AZD1981 (40 mg three times daily) or a placebo. A clinical assessment of UAS7 and ISS7 scores revealed a significant reduction in these scores when compared with the baseline scores before treatment. However, the primary endpoint (a reduction in UAS7 $\geq$ 9.5 points when compared with the baseline) was not achieved in this study. No significant differences were observed in terms of anti-histamines use or the frequency of angioedema-attacks between the treatment and control groups. No serious adverse events were observed and the overall treatment was well tolerated [52], Regarding biological effects, the treatment with AZD1981 significantly inhibited PGD2-mediated eosinophil migration to the skin. Despite failing to meet the primary endpoint, future studies evaluating the efficacy of AZD1981 with longer treatment duration and higher doses are needed.

4.3.2 Spleen tyrosine kinase (SYK) inhibitors

Spleen tyrosine kinase (SYK) is a pivotal player that regulates histamine release and the synthesis of immune mediators (e.g. leukotriene, prostaglandin) upon FcεRI activation in mast cells [55]. Nowadays, oral SYK inhibitors such as fostamatinib are used extensively in the treatment for autoimmune diseases such as immune thrombocytopenic purpura, chronic graft-versus-host disease and Rheumatoid Arthritis. A new intranasal SYK inhibitor, R112, was also proven to suppress FcεRI-related mediator release following mast cell degranulation, thereby suggesting that SYK inhibitors are extremely efficient in suppressing mast cell degranulation [56]. Based on the above data the use of SYK inhibitors to successfully treat CSU patients was not surprising. The first study to use SYK inhibitors was an in vitro study where a topical SYK inhibitor, was used in an ex vivo human skin model, GSK2646264. In this study it was shown that this inhibitor blocked the histamine release from mast cells through IgE signaling [57]. Following this study, a randomized, placebo-controlled phase I trial (NCT02424799) was conducted in order to evaluate the efficacy and safety of GSK2646264 0.5% and 1% topical cream in patients with CSU and cold urticarial. The results of this study are not available yet. In another in vitro study, the expression level of SYK was evaluated in mast cells from CSU patients. These patients were categorized according to the clinical out- come as responders and non-responders; the degree of basophil's histamine release and the expression of SYK protein in mast cells. This study found that the SYK protein was expressed significantly higher in responders when compared with non-responders and healthy controls. It also revealed that the increased expression of SYK was correlated with the spontaneous histamine release from mast cells in these patients [58].

4.4 Cytokine inhibitors

4.4.1 Anti IL-1

The IL-1 cytokine family in general and IL-1α and IL-1β, specifically have pro-inflammatory effects, which are neutralized by using the IL-1R antagonist. [59]. Several IL-1 mutations (NLRP3 genes) are collectively defined as auto-inflammatory syndromes, which cause the increased secretion of IL-1β. This is associated with a heterogeneous syndrome (NLRP3-AID (consisting of familial cold autoinflammatory syndrome, Muckle–Wells syndrome, and chronic infantile neurological, cutaneous and articular syndrome. The urticarial-like rash is one of most common hallmarks of these syndromes [60, 61]. IL-1 inhibitors, such as canakinumab (monoclonal antibody against of IL-1β), anakinra (recombinant IL-1R antagonist), and rilonacept (IL-1α/β blocker) are very effective in reducing inflammation and the clinical spectrum of these syndromes [62]. It is worth mentioning, that the emerging knowledge regarding the use of IL-1-blocking agents in the treatment of Schnitzler's syndrome, is characterized by the presence of urticarial rash and systemic inflammation [63, 64]. In on-going clinical trials, the effectiveness and safety of RPH-104 (a novel molecule against IL-1β), rilonacept, and canakinumab has been confirmed in Schnitzler syndrome (NCT04213274), acquired cold-contact urticaria (NCT02171416), and CSU (NCT01635127). The results of these trials have not yet been published. In few sporadic reports, anti-IL-1drugs were shown to be beneficial in CSU patients, who remained resistant to all classical therapies for CSU [65]. A new somatic mutation in NLRP3 was recently reported in two elderly patients with long-standing, refractory CSU associated with fever and increased CRP. Both of these patients improved dramatically following the usage of anakinra. As a result, it is assumed assumed that in patients with refractory urticaria and markers of systemic inflammation (a possible underlying NLRP3-related disorder), anti-IL-1 treatment requires further evaluation [66].

4.4.2 Anti-IL-4/13

In the process of Th2 differentiation several cytokines are produced. The most important cytokines in this process are interleukin-4 and IL-13 [59]. Dupilumab, a new monoclonal antibody directed against the alpha subunit of IL-4 and IL-13 receptors, was recently approved for the treatment of asthma, nasal polyposis, and atopic dermatitis [67]. Increased levels of IL-4 were recently demonstrated in patients with CSU, thereby suggesting a pathogenic role of both Th1/Th2 responses and raising the option of treating CSU with Dupilumab [68]. A recent case report involving six patients with concomitant atopic dermatitis and CSU who were refractory to high dose of omalizumab (600 mg\4 weeks) documented their successful treated with Dupilumab. In this report, it was postulated that the beneficial therapeutic effect of Dupilumab could be the result of its blocking Th2 inflammatory pathways by inhibiting IL-4 and IL-13, respective [69]. Currently, there are three ongoing, phase II/III clinical studies investigating the efficacy and safety of Dupilumab in CSU (NCT03749135, NCT04180488 (EFC16461-CUPID)) and cholinergic urticaria (NCT03749148) unresponsive to a high dosage of antihistamines and omalizumab.

4.4.3 Anti IL-5

Eosinophils, are considered to have a pivotal role in the pathogenesis of CSU. Many reports have demonstrated elevated numbers of eosinophils in urticarial lesions when compared with normal skin. Their contribution to CSU pathogenesis is probably achieved through interactions with mast cells, the secretion of histamine and other inflammatory mediators and the activation of the coagulation cascade [70]. The important role of interleukin-5 (IL-5) in eosinophil development and maturation, as well as in increased chemotaxis towards skin urticarial lesions has been well documented [59]. Several monoclonal antibodies were recently approved for the treatment of eosinophil related airway diseases (e.g. asthma, Churg-Strauss syndrome, nasal polyposis etc.) by targeting IL-5 (reslizumab, mepolizumab) or its receptor, IL-5R (benralizumab). These drugs were recently used in three CSU patients who were refractory to classical therapies; two patients responded well and showed a significant improvement with Reslizumab and mepolizumab [71, 72], while the other patient who suffered from symptomatic dermographism (SD) benefited from their treatment with benralizumab [73]. In a recent single-blind, repeated measures study, 12 CSU patients were treated with benralizumab (30 mg subcutaneously) every 4 weeks for 12 weeks following a single dose of a placebo. Among the nine patients who completed the study, five had complete response. Their UAS7 and CU-Q2oL scores improved significantly with benralizumab when compared with the placebo [74]. Gene-expression analysis in patients with CSU following benralizumab treatment demonstrated the normalization of SIGLEC-8 expression and IL-4/5 induced inflammation [75]. Although the results imply that eosinophils play a role in CSU, the exact mechanism of action has not yet been understood. Two clinical trials investigating the efficacy of benralizumab

(NCT03183024) and mepolizumab (NCT03494881) in CSU are still in progress, and their results are not yet available. Regarding benralizumab, a phase IIb study (ARROYO Trial- D3259C00001) is set to start soon.

5. Potential therapeutic approaches

5.1 Eosinophils, mast cells, basophils

5.1.1 Siglec-8

The Siglecs are a family of sialic-acid-binding immunoglobulin-like lectins, which are thought to promote cell–cell interactions and regulate the functions of cells in the innate and adaptive immune systems through glycan recognition. These proteins have regulatory effects on intercellular and intracellular signaling such as the inhibition of cellular proliferation/activation and the induction of apoptosis [76, 77]. Siglec-8 is highly and selectively expressed by eosinophils, but it became clear that it is also expressed by human mast cells and weakly, but consistently, by human basophils. Studies showed that the activation of Siglec-8 induces eosinophil apoptosis (in a caspase-, mitochondrial-, and reactive oxygen species–dependent way). It was also shown that activated eosinophils are especially sensitive to Siglec-8-induced death [78]. It also inhibits the release of FcεRI-mediated histamine and PGD2 from mast cells [79, 80]. In a recent phase I, randomized, placebo-controlled study conducted with more than 50 healthy volunteers, a single dose of a monoclonal anti-Siglec-8 antibody, namely- AK002 (autolimab) (0.001, 0.003, 0.01, 0.03, 0.1, 0.3, and 1 mg/kg IV), resulted in the complete depletion of circulating eosinophils within one hour from the infusion. This effect was maintained for up to 84 days only in the group who received 1 mg/kg. This result pointed to a possible administration schedule of AK002 at monthly or quarterly intervals [81]. Additionally, in another additional study it was also demonstrated that treatment with AK002 provided symptomatic and histologic improvement in patients with eosinophilic esophagitis [82]. Taking this into consideration, a phase IIa study in CSU and CIndU (cholinergic urticaria and symptomatic dermographism) patients was conducted. These patients received six doses of AK002. At week 22, following treatment, based on changes in UCT score - the response rates in CSU patients were the following, complete + partial response in 92% and 86% in omalizumab-naive (n = 14) and omalizumab refractory (n = 12) patients, respectively. In the 12-month open-label extension phase, the response was sustained. No adverse events were observed, with only mild-to-moderate infusion-related reactions recorded [83, 84]. These results suggest that in the future, anti-Siglec-8 antibodies might be a treatment option for CSU patients, who are either omalizumab naïve or refractory to omalizumab.

5.1.2 Other molecules (SHIP-1, PI3K, CD200)

Many new regulatory molecules are recently evaluated for their potential inhibitory effect on mast cell degranulation. Some of them are under development and are to be included in the pipe-line of clinical trials for the treatment of CSU. Among these molecules are SHIP and CD200R, which deserve our attention. It has been shown that SHIP-negative mast cells are more likely to degranulate following IgE binding [85]. The inhibitory effects of SHIP-1 occur through the hydrolysis of phosphatidylinositol 3, 4, 5-trisphosphate by limiting the entry of extracellular calcium, thereby decreasing phosphoinositide 3-kinase (PI3K)-mediated mast cell activation [86–88]. CD200R is a member of the Ig supergene family that is primarily expressed on myeloid cells. In vivo studies demonstrated that CD200R is an inhibitory receptor that is capable of regulating the activation threshold of inflammatory immune responses. Furthermore, CD200R was also shown to be expressed on mouse and human mast cells and that engagement of CD200R by agonist Abs or ligand results in a potent inhibition of mast cell degranulation and cytokine secretion responses. The proposed mechanism for that effect was possibly due to the inhibition of FcεRI activation that was observed both in vitro and in vivo. [88] Considering their regulatory functions on mast cells, the use of SHIP, CD200R antibodies, or PI3K inhibitors for the treatment of CSU is of great interest.

5.1.3 Anti-histamine H4 receptor

The emerging field of histamine H4 receptors in allergy and clinical immunology is continuously growing. H4 histamine receptor, is a member of the G protein-coupled receptor superfamily that is largely expressed in haematopoietic cells and plays an increasing role in the regulation of immune responses. H4 receptors modulate eosinophil migration and selective recruitment of mast cells that leads to an increased histamine-release and chronic inflammation. It is also involved in T cell differentiation thereby is involved in many immunomodulatory pathways. The observation that H4 is a histamine receptor on many immune cells shed light on the potential of their targeting in inflammatory disorders, such as allergy, chronic pruritus and autoimmune diseases e.g. CSU [89]. Several ongoing clinical studies currently taking place are aimed at evaluating the beneficial effect of targeting H4 receptors in patients suffering from atopic dermatitis and pruritus (JNJ-7777120, ZPL-3893787). Preliminary results have indicated a significant reduction in histamine-mediated scratch and Th2-induced inflammation in atopic dermatitis [90, 91]. These results are encouraging and indicate the need to further evaluate any potential benefits of these drugs in the treatment of CSU.

5.1.4 Mas-related gene X2

MrgX2 is a member of Mas-related genes that is primarily expressed in human dorsal root ganglia and mast cells and is activated by basic peptides. MrgX2 is a multi-ligand receptor responding to various exogenous and endogenous stimuli. As they are highly expressed on skin mast cells, MRGPRX2 triggers their degranulation and release of pro inflammatory mediators, thus promoting multicellular signaling cascades, such as itch induction and transmission in sensory neurons. The expression of MRGPRX2 by skin mast cells and the levels of the MRGPRX2 agonists (eg, substance P, major basic protein, eosinophil peroxidase) are up-regulated in the serum and skin of patients with inflammatory and pruritic skin diseases, such as CSU and atopic dermatitis. Thus, MRGPRX2 and its agonists might possibly be potential biomarkers for the progression of cutaneous inflammatory diseases and the response to treatment in the future. In addition, they may well represent promising targets for the prevention and treatment of signs and symptoms in patients with skin diseases or drug reactions [92].

6. Anti-IgE, B cells

6.1 Quilizimab

Quilizumab, is another new humanized monoclonal antibody directed specifically against membrane-bound IgE. This molecule was also evaluated for its efficacy and safety for the treatment of CSU in a phase II trial. Unfortunately, following a 20-week treatment with quilizumab 450 mg or a placebo every 4 weeks, no statistically significant differences were observed in all clinical scores ISS7, HSS7, and UAS7 – between the two groups. Moreover, even in the minimally important difference (MID) range the quilizumab group also failed to attain significant differences. [93]. Thus, further development of quilizumab for CSU was discontinued.

6.2 T cell related therapies

6.2.1 TSLP

The expression of thymic stromal lymphopoietin (TSLP), a promotor of Th2 response, was proven to be increased in patients with CSU, thus making the anti-TSLP monoclonal antibody, tezepelumab, a potential treatment alternative for CSU [94, 95].

6.2.2 Anti-IL-17

The finding of increased blood levels of IL-17 in CSU patients was previously reported to be in association with CSU severity. This encouraged us to assess the status of IL-17 in the skin of CSU patients, thus, demonstrating increased IL-17 expression in CD4+ T cells and mast cells of both lesional and non-lesional skin of severe CSU patients. With this in mind, eight severe CSU patients (refractory to all approved therapies and steroid dependent) were treated with the anti-IL-17A antibody, secukinumab, demonstrating a significant improvement in CSU disease activity and were able to discontinue steroids. Future studies should be planned in order to expand this promising therapeutic approach [16, 96].

7. Summary

The need for new treatments evolve from the fact that 15–20% of severe CSU patients will stay unresponsive to Omalizumab and are defined as being of un-met needs. Thus, a better understanding of the complexity of CSU pathogenesis led to the development of many new treatment options. In this chapter we reviewed the known and the ongoing clinical studies of the new treatments for severe CSU. We expect that some of these strategies will be efficient and will be added to the market of the existing therapies.

Author details

Zahava Vadasz [1*] and Elias Toubi[2]

1 Bnai-Zion Medical Center, Rappaport Faculty of Medicine, Technion, Haifa, Israel

2 Holy-Family Hospital, Nazareth, Israel

*Address all correspondence to: zahava.vadas@b-zion.org.il

References

[1] Lapi F, Cassano N, Pegoraro V, Cataldo N, Heiman F, Cricelli I, et al. Epidemiology of chronic spontaneous urticaria: results from a nationwide, population-based study in Italy. Br J Dermatol 2016; 174: 996-1004.

[2] Toubi E, Kessel A, Avshovich N, Bamberger E, Sabo E, Nusem D, Panasoff J. Clinical and laboratory parameters in predicting chronic urticarial duration: a prospective study of 139 patients. Allergy 2004; 59: 869-73.

[3] Stepaniuk P, Manstein K, Kanani A. Natural history, prognostic factors and patient perceived response to treatment in chronic spontaneous urticaria. Allergy Asthma Clin Immunol 2020; 16: 63.

[4] Erol K, Ertas SK, Ertas R. Fatigue is common and predicted by female gender and sleep disturbance in patients with chronic spontaneous urticaria. J Allergy Clin Immunol Pract 2021; 9: 469-476.

[5] Staubach P, Dechene M, Metz M, Magerl M, Siebenhaar F, Weller k, et al. High prevalence of mental disorders and emotional distress in patients with chronic spontaneous urticaria. Acta Derm Venereol 2011; 91: 557-61.

[6] Kolkhir P, Pogorelov D, Olisova O, Maurer M. Comorbidity and pathogenic links of chronic spontaneous urticaria and systemic lupus erythematosus-a systemic review. Clin Exp Allergy 2016; 46: 275-87.

[7] Ghazanfar MN, Kibsgaard L, Thomsen SF, Vestergaard C. Risk of comorbidities in patients diagnosed with chronic urticaria: A nationwide registry-study. World Allergy Organ J 2020; 13: 100097.

[8] Sanchez-Borges M, Capriles-Hulett A, Caballero-Fonseca F, Gonzalez-Aveledo L. Biomarkers of treatment efficacy in patients with chronic spontaneous urticaria. Eur Ann Allergy Clin Immunol 2018; 50: 5-9.

[9] Kolkhir P, Andre F, Church MK, Metz M. Potential blood biomarkers in chronic spontaneous urticaria. Clin Exp Allergy 2017; 47: 19-36.

[10] Vestergaard C, Toubi E, Maurer M, Triggiani M, Ballmer-Weber B, Marsland A, et al. Treatment of chronic spontaneous urticarial with an inadequate response to H1-antihistamines: an expert opinion. Eur J Dermatol 2017; 27: 10-19.

[11] Mekori YA, Giorno RC, Anderson P, Kohler PF. Lymphocyte subpopulations in the skin of patients with chronic urticaria. J Allergy Clin Immunol 1983; 72: 681-84.

[12] Toubi E, Adir-Shani A, Kessel A, Shmuel Z, Sabo E, Hacham H. Immune aberrations in B and T lymphocytes derived from chronic urticaria patients. J Clin Immunol 2000;20(5):371-378.

[13] Chen Q, Zhong H, Chen WC, Zhai Z, Zhou Z, Song Z, Hao F. Different expression patterns of plasma Th1, Th2, Th17 and Th22-related cytokines correlate with serum auto-reactivity and allergen sensitivity in chronic spontaneous urticaria. J Eur Acad Dermatol Venerol 2018; 32: 441-48.

[14] Feng H, Feng J, Zhang Z, Xu Q, Hu M, Wu Y, Lu Y. Role of IL-9 and IL-10 in the pathogenesis of chronic spontaneous urticarial through the JAK/STAT signaling pathway. Cell Biochem Fuct 2020; 38: 480-89.

[15] Auyeung P, Mittag D, Hodgkin PD, Harrison LC. Autoreactive T cells in chronic spontaneous urticarial target the IgE Fc receptor Iα subunit. J Allergy Clin Immunol 2016; 138:761-68.

[16] Sabag DA, Matanes L, Bejar J, Sheffer H, Barzilai A, Church MK, et al. Interleukin-17 is a potential player and treatment target in severe chronic spontaneous urticaria. Clin Exp Allergy 2020; 50: 799-804.

[17] Bracken SJ, Abraham S, Macleod AS. Autoimmune theories of chronic urticaria. Front Immunol 2019; 10:627.

[18] Kolkhir P, Church MK, Weller K, Metz M, Schmetzer O, Maurer M. Autoimmune chronic spontaneous urticarial: what we know and what we do not know. J Allergy Clin Immunol 2017; 139: 1772-81.

[19] Altrichter S, Zampeli V, Ellrich A, Zhang Ke, Church MK, Maurer M. IgM and IgA addition to IgG autoantibodies against FcRI are frequent and associated with disease markers of chronic spontaneous urticaria. Allergy 2020; doi: 10.1111.

[20] Church MK, Kolkhir P, Metz M, Maurer M. The role and relevance of mast cells in urticaria. Immunol Rev 2018; 282: 232-47.

[21] Ferrer M. Immunological events in chronic spontaneous urticaria. Clin Transl Allergy 2015; 5:30.

[22] Altrichter S, Frischbutter S, Fok JS, Kolkhir P, Jiao Q, Skov PS, et al. The role of eosinophils in chronic spontaneous urticaria. J Allergy Clin Immunol 2020; doi: 10.1016.

[23] Guillen-Aguinaga S, Jauregui P, Auinaga-Ontoso E, Guillen-Grima F, Ferre M. Up dosing nonsedating antihistamines in patients with chronic spontaneous urticarial: a systemic review and meta-analysis. Br J Dermatol 2016; 175: 1153-65.

[24] Fradin MS, Ellis CN, Goldfarb MT, Voorhees JJ. Oral cyclosporine for severe chronic idiopathic urticaria and angioedema. J Am Acad Dermatol 1991; 25: 1065-7.

[25] Toubi E, Blant A, Kessel A, Golan TD. Low-dose cyclosporine A in the treatment of severe chronic idiopathic urticaria. Allergy 1997; 52: 312-6.

[26] Vena GA, Cassano N, Colombo D, Peruzzi E, Piggato P. Cyclosporine in chronic idiopathic urticaria: a double-blind, randomized, placebo-controlled trial. J Am Acad Dermatol 2006; 55: 705-9.

[27] Kulthanan K, Chaweekulrat P, Komoltri C, Hunnangkul S, Tuchinda P, Chularojanamontri L, Maurer M. Cyclosporine for chronic spontaneous urticaria: A meta-analysis and systemic review. J Allergy Clin Immunol Pract 2018; 6: 586-99.

[28] Kulthanan K, Subchookul C, Hunnangkul S, Chularojanamontri L, Tuchinda P. Factors predicting the response to cyclosporine treatment in patients with chronic spontaneous urticaria: a systemic review. Allergy Asthma Immunol Res 2019; 11: 736-55.

[29] Saini SS, Bindslev-Jensen C, Maurer M, Grob LJ, Baskan EB, Bradley MS, et al. Efficacy and safety of omalizumab in patients with chronic idiopathic/spontaneous urticarial who remain symptomatic on H1 anti-histamines: a randomized, placebo-controlled study. J Invest Dermatol 2015; 135: 67-75.

[30] Zuberbier T, Aberer W, Asero R, Abdol-Latiff AH, Baker D, Ballmer-Weber B, et al. The EAACI/GA2LEN/WAO guideline for the definition, classification, diagnosis and management of urticaria. Allergy 2018; 73: 1393-1414.

[31] Chang TW, Chen C, Lin CJ, Metz M, Church MK, Maurer M. The potential pharmacologic mechanisms of omalizumab in patients with chronic spontaneous urticaria. J Allergy Clin Immunol 2015; 135: 337-42.

[32] Magen E, Chikovani T, Waitman DA, Kahan N. Factors related to omalizumab resistance in chronic spontaneous urticaria. Allergy Asthma Proc 2019; 40: 273-78.

[33] Metz M, Vadasz Z, Kocaturk E, Gimenez-Arnau AMK. Omalizumab updosing in chronic spontaneous urticarial: an overview of real world evidence. Clin Rev Allergy Immunol 2020; 59: 38-45.

[34] Gasser P, Tarchevskaya SS, Guntern P, Brigger D, Ruppli R, Zbären N, et al. The mechanistic and functional profile of the therapeutic anti-IgE antibody ligelizumab differs from omalizumab. Nat Commun. 2020;11:165.

[35] Arm JP, Bottoli I, Skerjanec A, Floch D, Groenewegen A, Maahs S, et al. Pharmacokinetics, pharmacodynamics and safety of QGE031 (ligelizumab), a novel high-affinity anti-IgE antibody, in atopic subjects. Clin Exp Allergy. 2014;44:1371-85.

[36] Maurer M, Giménez-Arnau AM, Sussman G, Metz M, Baker DR, Bauer A, et al. Ligelizumab for chronic spontaneous urticaria. N Engl J Med. 2019;381:1321-32.

[37] Soong W, Bernstein J, Sussman G, Lanier B, Sitz K, Maurer M, et al. Long-term treatment with ligelizumab achieves prolonged symptom control during the post-treatment follow-up. J Allergy Clin Immunol. 2020;145:AB341.

[38] Sitz K, Soong W, Lanier B, Kobayashi K, Barve A, Hua E, et al. P153 ligelizumab reduces rescue medication use in patients with chronic spontaneous urticaria: phase 2b study results. Ann Allergy Asthma Immunol. 2019;123:S28.

[39] Soong W, Lanier B, Sitz K, Kobayashi K, Barve A, Hua E, et al. P151 ligelizumab achieves sustained control of angioedema in patients with chronic spontaneous urticaria. Ann Allergy Asthma Immunol. 2019;123:S27.

[40] Giménez-Arnau A M., Salman A. Targeted Therapy for Chronic Spontaneous Urticaria: Rationale and Recent Progress. Drugs 2020;80: 1617-1634.

[41] Cohen S, Tuckwell K, Katsumoto TR, Zhao R, Galanter J, Lee C, et al. Fenebrutinib versus placebo or adalimumab in rheumatoid arthritis: a randomized, double-blind, phase II Trial (ANDES Study). Arthritis Rheumatol. 2020. https://doi.org/10.1002/art.41275.

[42] Angst D, Gessier F, Janser P, Vulpetti A, Wälchli R, Beerli C, et al. Discovery of LOU064 (Remibrutinib), a potent and highly selective covalent inhibitor of Bruton's Tyrosine Kinase. J Med Chem. 2020;63:5102-18.

[43] Wedi B. Bruton tyrosine kinase inhibition in dermatology and allergology. Hautarzt. 2018;69:519-22.

[44] Smiljkovic D, Blatt K, Stefanzl G, Dorofeeva Y, Skrabs C, Focke-Tejkl M, et al. BTK inhibition is a potent approach to block IgE-mediated histamine release in human basophils. Allergy. 2017;72: 1666-76.

[45] Gabizon R, London N. A fast and clean BTK inhibitor. J Med Chem. 2020;63:5100-1.

[46] Marshall MJE, Stopforth RJ, Cragg MS. Therapeutic antibodies: what have we learnt from targeting CD20 and where are we going? Front Immunol. 2017;8:1245.

[47] Mallipeddi R, Grattan CEH. Lack of response of severe steroid dependent chronic urticaria to rituximab. Clin Exp Dermatol. 2007;32:333-4.

[48] Arkwright PD. Anti-CD20 or anti-IgE therapy for severe chronic autoimmune urticaria. J Allergy Clin Immunol. 2009;123:510-1.

[49] Chakravarty SD, Yee AF, Paget SA. Rituximab successfully treats refractory

chronic autoimmune urticaria caused by IgE receptor autoantibodies. J Allergy Clin Immunol. 2011;128:1354-5.

[50] Steinweg S, Gaspari A. Rituximab for the treatment of recalcitrant chronic autoimmune urticaria. J Drugs Dermatol. 2015;14:1387.

[51] Combalia A, Losno RA, Prieto-González S, Mascaró JM. Rituximab in refractory chronic spontaneous urticaria: an encouraging therapeutic approach. Skin Pharmacol Physiol. 2018;31:184-7.

[52] Oliver ET, Chichester K, Devine K, Sterba PM, Wegner C, Vonakis BM, et al. Effects of an oral CRTh2 antagonist (AZD1981) on eosinophil activity and symptoms in chronic spontaneous urticaria. Int Arch Allergy Immunol. 2019;179:21-30.

[53] Palikhe NS, Kim SH, Ye YM, Hur GY, Cho BY, Park HS. Association of CRTH2 gene polymorphisms with the required dose of antihistamines in patients with chronic urticaria. Pharmacogenomics. 2009;10:375-83.

[54] Oliver ET, Sterba PM, Devine K, Vonakis BM, Saini SS. Altered expression of chemoattractant receptor-homologous molecule expressed on TH2 cells on blood basophils and eosinophils in patients with chronic spontaneous urticaria. J Allergy Clin Immunol. 2016; 137(304-306):e1.

[55] Altman K, Chang C. Pathogenic intracellular and autoimmune mechanisms in urticaria and angioedema. Clin Rev Allergy Immunol. 2013;45: 47-62.

[56] Rossi A, Herlaar E, Braselmann S, Huynh S, Taylor V, Frances R, et al. Identification of the Syk kinase inhibitor R112 by a human mast cell screen [Internet]. J Allergy Clin Immunol 2006;118:749-55.

[57] Ramirez Molina C, Falkencrone S, Skov PS, Hooper-Greenhill E, Barker M, Dickson MC. GSK2646264, a spleen tyrosine kinase inhibitor, attenuates the release of histamine in ex vivo human skin. Br J Pharmacol. 2019;176:1135-42.

[58] Saini SS, Paterniti M, Vasagar K, Gibbsons SP Jr, Patricia M, Vonakis BM. Cultured peripheral blood mast cells from chronic idiopathic urticaria patients spontaneously degranulate upon IgE sensitization: relationship to expression of Syk and SHIP-2. Clin Immunol. 2009;132:342-8.

[59] Akdis M, Aab A, Altunbulakli C, Azkur K, Costa RA, Crameri R, et al. Interleukins (from IL-1 to IL-38), interferons, transforming growth factor β, and TNF-α: receptors, functions, and roles in diseases. J Allergy Clin Immunol. 2016;138:984-1010.

[60] Wang D, Duncan B, Li X, Shi J. The role of NLRP3 inflammasome in infection-related, immune-mediated and autoimmune skin diseases. J Dermatol Sci. 2020;98:146-51.

[61] Krause K, Metz M, Makris M, Zuberbier T, Maurer M. The role of interleukin-1 in allergy-related disorders. Curr Opin Allergy Clin Immunol. 2012;12:477-84.

[62] Federici S, Martini A, Gattorno M. The central role of anti-IL-1 blockade in the treatment of monogenic and multi-factorial autoinflammatory diseases. Front Immunol. 2013;4:351.

[63] Krause K, Mahamed A, Weller K, Metz M, Zuberbier T, Maurer M. Efficacy and safety of canakinumab in urticarial vasculitis: an open-label study. J Allergy Clin Immunol. 2013;132:751-4.

[64] Néel A, Henry B, Barbarot S, Masseau A, Perrin F, Bernier C, et al. Long-term effectiveness and safety of interleukin-1 receptor antagonist (anakinra) in Schnitzler's syndrome:

A french multicenter study. Autoimmun Rev. 2014;13:1035-41.

[65] Bodar EJ, Simon A, De Visser M, Van Der Meer JWM. Complete remission of severe idiopathic cold urticaria on interleukin-1 receptor antagonist (anakinra). Neth J Med. 2009;67:302-5.

[66] Assrawi E, Louvrier C, Lepelletier C, Georgin-Lavialle S, Bouaziz JD, Awad F, et al. Somatic mosaic NLRP3 mutations and inflammasome activation in late-onset chronic urticaria. J Invest Dermatol. 2020;140:791-8.

[67] Hendricks AJ, Yosipovitch G, Shi VY. Dupilumab use in dermatologic conditions beyond atopic dermatitis—a systematic review. J Dermatolog Treat. 2019 (ahead of print).

[68] Ferrer M, Luquin E, Sanchez-Ibarrola A, Moreno C, Sanz ML, Kaplan AP. Secretion of cytokines, histamine and leukotrienes in chronic urticaria. Int Arch Allergy Immunol. 2002;129:254-60.

[69] Lee JK, Simpson RS. Dupilumab as a novel therapy for difficult to treat chronic spontaneous urticaria. J Allergy Clin Immunol Pract. 2019;7(1659-1661):e1.

[70] Altrichter S, Frischbutter S, Fok JS, Kolkhir P, Jiao Q, Skov PS, et al. The role of eosinophils in chronic spontaneous urticaria. J Allergy Clin Immunol. 2020 (ahead of print).

[71] Maurer M, Altrichter S, Metz M, Zuberbier T, Church MK, Bergmann KC. Benefit from reslizumab treatment in a patient with chronic spontaneous urticaria and cold urticaria. J Eur Acad Dermatol Venereol. 2018;32:e112–e11313.

[72] Magerl M, Terhorst D, Metz M, Altrichter S, Zuberbier T, Maurer M, et al. Benefit of mepolizumab treatment in a patient with chronic spontaneous urticaria. J Dtsch Dermatol Ges. 2018; 16:477-8.

[73] Bergmann KC, Altrichter S, Maurer M. Benefit of benralizumab treatment in a patient with chronic symptomatic dermographism. J Eur Acad Dermatol Venereol. 2019;33: e413–e415415.

[74] Singh U, Bernstein J. Clinical efficacy of benralizumab and its role in modifying mechanistic pathways in chronic idiopathic urticaria refractory to H1-antagonists. J Allergy Clin Immunol. 2020;145:AB249.

[75] Singh U, Bernstein J. Demonstrating clinical efficacy of benralizumab in chronic spontaneous urticaria via normalization of gene-expression in biological samples. J Allergy Clin Immunol. 2020;145:AB340.

[76] Crocker PR, Paulson JC, Varki A. Siglecs and their roles in the immune system. Nat Rev Immunol. 2007;7:255-66.

[77] O'Sullivan JA, Chang AT, Youngblood BA, Bochner BS. Eosinophil and mast cell Siglecs: from biology to drug target. J Leukoc Biol. 2020;108: 73-81.

[78] von Gunten S, Bochner BS. Basic and clinical immunology of Siglecs. Ann N Y Acad Sci. 2008;1143:61-82.

[79] Bochner BS. Siglec-8 on human eosinophils and mast cells, and Siglec-F on murine eosinophils, are functionally related inhibitory receptors. Clin Exp Allergy. 2009;39:317-24.

[80] Kiwamoto T, Kawasaki N, Paulson J, Bochner B. Siglec-8 as a drugable target to treat eosinophil and mast cell-associated conditions. Pharmacol Ther. 2012;135: 327-36.

[81] Rasmussen HS, Chang AT, Tomasevic N, Bebbington C. A randomized, double-blind, placebo-controlled, ascending dose Phase 1 study of AK002, a novel Siglec-8 selective monoclonal antibody, in

healthy subjects. J Allergy Clin Immunol. 2018;141:AB403.

[82] Hirano I, Peterson K, Murray J, Dellon E, Falk G, Gonsalves N, et al. AK002, an Anti-Siglec-8 antibody, depletes tissue eosinophils and improves dysphagia symptoms in patients with eosinophilic esophagitis. J Allergy Clin Immunol. 2020;145:AB167.

[83] Altrichter S, Staubach P, Pasha M, Rasmussen H, Singh B, Chang A, et al. P152 clinical activity of Ak002, an anti-siglec-8 antibody, in multiple forms of uncontrolled chronic urticaria. Ann Allergy Asthma Immunol. 2019;123: S27–S2828.

[84] Altrichter S, Staubach P, Pasha M, Rasmussen H, Singh B, Chang A, et al. Clinical activity of AK002, an anti-siglec-8 monoclonal antibody, in treatment-refractory chronic urticaria. J Allergy Clin Immunol. 2020;145:AB239.

[85] Huber M, Helgason CD, Damen JE, Liu L, Humphries RK, Krystal G. The src homology 2-containing inositol phosphatase (SHIP) is the gatekeeper of mast cell degranulation. Proc Natl Acad Sci USA. 1998;95:11330-5.

[86] Gimborn K, Lessmann E, Kuppig S, Krystal G, Huber M. SHIP down-regulates FcεR1-induced degranulation at supraoptimal IgE or antigen levels. J Immunol. 2005;136:4565-72.

[87] Kim M-S, Rådinger M, Gilfillan AM. The multiple roles of phosphoinositide 3-kinase in mast cell biology. Trends Immunol. 2008;29:493-501.

[88] Cherwinski HM, Murphy CA, Joyce BL, Bigler ME, Song YS, Zurawski SM, et al. The CD200 receptor is a novel and potent regulator of murine and human mast cell function. J Immunol. 2005;174:1348-56.

[89] Zampeli E, Tiligada E. The role of histamine H 4 receptor in immune and inflammatory disorders. Br J Pharmacol. 2009;157:24-33.

[90] Cowden JM, Zhang M, Dunford PJ, Thurmond RL. The histamine H4 receptor mediates inflammation and pruritus in Th2-dependent dermal inflammation. J Invest Dermatol. 2010; 130:1023-33.

[91] Thurmond RL. The histamine H4 receptor: from orphan to the clinic. Front Pharmacol. 2015;6:1-11.

[92] Fujisawa D, Kashiwakura J-I, Kita H, Kikukawa Y, Fujitani Y, Sasaki-Sakamoto T, et al. Expression of Mas-related gene X2 on mast cells is upregulated in the skin of patients with severe chronic urticaria. J Allergy Clin Immunol. 2014;134(622-633):e9.

[93] Harris JM, Cabanski CR, Scheerens H, Samineni D, Bradley MS, Cochran C, et al. A randomized trial of quilizumab in adults with refractory chronic spontaneous urticaria. J Allergy Clin Immunol. 2016;138:1730-2.

[94] Kay AB, Clark P, Maurer M, Ying S. Elevations in T-helper- 2-initiating cytokines (interleukin-33, interleukin-25 and thymic stromal lymphopoietin) in lesional skin from chronic spontaneous ('idiopathic') urticaria. Br J Dermatol. 2015;172:1294-302.

[95] Takai T. TSLP expression: cellular sources, triggers, and regulatory mechanisms. Allergol Int. 2012;61:3-17.

[96] Toubi E, Vadasz Z. The Emerging Role of IL-17 in the Immune-Pathogenesis of Chronic Spontaneous Urticaria. Immunotargets Ther. 2020 Oct 22;9: 217-223. doi: 10.2147/ITT.S266410. eCollection 2020.